AF254721

Living Healthy Made Easy

ISRAA HILLES

Copyright © 2021 Israa Hilles

All rights reserved.

ISBN: 978-1-7776579-1-8

Contents

Chapter 1; Emotion and Eating

Every day, you gather insight, pleasant or unpleasant, painful at times... and create the man and the woman you are today. Your body is essential because it preserves you, protects you, it represents your mood.

As a teenager, you have become tiny, and you have through the years been completed and no longer know the girl or the child you recall – a carnal recollection – a memory filtered through years of struggle with life activities, weight, and self.

As a youth, you see yourself playing sports with your peers every day, filled with enthusiasm and pleasure in living, convinced that all of your projects will be implemented and that this young athletic and charismatic guy can continue. What changed in 20 years? What happened?

What are the methods used to gain or lose weight over the years?

The function of emotions in the body's transformation

Communication of the heart and brain

This is a two-way conversation.

The body absorbs from the outside messages (stimulus) and converts them into sensations, positions, languages, ideas, feelings, choices. Your brain converts stimuli that the body perceives into feelings, ideas, and languages simultaneously.

If your brain is anxious, your body would be restless. This may be helpful since tension helps the body to warn of imminent threats and mobilize the requisite resources for your well-being. Long exposure in a stress situation, on the other side, has adverse consequences on the body.

Effective heart communication — the brain results in a careful equilibrium between the body's capacity to respond, mobilize muscle energy, and relax, rebuild, and render accessible points. This is the independent nervous system's function: Allowing the body to react to the surroundings in real-time. If you can supply the required energy at once and replenish it in adequate quantities, adaptation is optimum.

The scientific term describing this concept of equilibrium between capital and energy spending is the homeostasis or preservation of internal (health) security in an unpredictable climate.

If this internal condition is imbalanced, the organism weakens and produces more or less harmful diseases for its life.

Weight and conduct

Weight challenges are due to unbalanced diets, but most often because of shifts in the body structure. Destructive emotions, including frustration, fear, disappointment, resentment, and sorrow, tend to be driving factors. More frequently, experiences in infancy that may have been linked with an emotion and a diet need to be used.

The core is the emotional center: It is directly linked to the limbic brain, a dynamic region.

One philosophy describes the six basic emotions: pleasure, sorrow, terror, wrath, disgust, and surprise. Secondary or combined emotions are a combination of fundamental emotions: Shame, for instance, is a blend of fear and rage.

Some ideas, such as those of social appraisal, reflect a wider variety of feelings with knowledge and other individual needs.

When a lousy emotion hurts you, you prefer to curl up to be protected or to behave, attack, or run as your reptile brain or primal brain dictates.

The Latin root of the term "emotion" that is "ex-mover" or "to move outwardly" reminds us of its importance: The feeling will then require a behavior. If the surface is pessimistic and goes on for a time, the action can be disproportionate, inappropriate, or even contradictory. Wouldn't you be shocked to consume any junk food when you're sad?

Will you render tension fat?

We need to distinguish between persistent stress or acute stress. The first would tend to get fat (increase in waist circumference). In contrast, the second would draw so much energy over a short period that the body, by an adaptation mechanism, would become lighter by burning calories.

Rage, for instance, is sending so much cortisol, the stress hormone, that its results are felt through the body for around 4 hours—higher cardiac and respiratory rhythm, blood flow, coagulation, and blood vessel vasoconstriction.

Cortisol is triggered by the autonomous nervous system's sympathetic "cardio-accelerating," which controls the body's entire automated and involuntary regulatory system, such as ventilation, digestion, energy generation, etc.

Under permanent cortisol, the adrenal glands get drained, and the body gets stressed. Metabolism stops and stores the body in the run-up to a potential episode of tension for fear of losing energy to avoid, battle, or escape for protection.

Intake of emotional food

Babies link to the world through food, through their mouths, throughout the first days of existence.

Mama loves breastfeeding infants so much that the baby's flesh will recall it even years later! Father wants to feed the kid so much that his baby registers the least of the sentimental memories.

Whether you have current or previous challenging encounters, the body can recall and intensify the physical and psychological manifestations if you enter the same condition much later. It is a means of protecting the organism that warns the body that a threat exists.

The Award

When you feed in reaction to an excessively intense emotion: Why? What's the echo in you? Why do you want to load anything with? And why will it be sweet or oily necessarily, or both? Why not broccoli steamed?

The sense of relaxation may be sensual, olfactory, factual, or dietary. When your mom comforted you as a kid of sweets, today you indeed have this reflection that will make you feel emotionally happy, in a bubble of reassuring sugar.

Responsibility of parents

Knowing all of this, any parent has a responsibility to be careful of what his child brings to adulthood by knowledge and vocabulary, including those not meant for him.

I see too many mothers or fathers parenting their little cod alone, complaining to him loudly about his anxieties, his feelings shifting, his inconsistencies. It's not tolerable!

Ensure the child remains away from your couple, your job, your everyday issues, your financial concerns, your friendship with your parents (so his grandparents): he has not asked something and maintains it as long as he can.

Words' Importance

Be cautious not to build a dependency on your child's emotions: If it's fair, the little "too much" encourages the kid to be placed on the same stage as an adult he loads with vacuum becomes unsafe and harmful for the child.

Did you get extra pounds? Do you think in your dynamic environment, they have their source? Could you not make your child hold them (ren)?

Take caution and consult to guarantee that the harmful thoughts do not transmit to a bit of being who has no resources or knowledge yet to comprehend.

Family Food, an Exchange and Connection Moment

Privilege meal times at the table, as much as practicable with the relatives, without distractions other than the other's eyes.

Don't push a starving kid anymore: We are not in French wartime, so make sure he maintains his innate capacity to claim, "Stop, I'm not hungry anymore!"

Take the time to feed, sample, and watch the food: Enjoy the time. Enjoy the moment.

Careful Hearing

Listen and monitor your kid, as something affects his behavior, food, or otherwise, and allow it the ability to discharge each phase in life emotionally.

Werkzeuge for the kid

Cardiac coherence, which synchronizes the cardiovascular, body, and mind, is a validated and playful protocol for developing concentration, understanding, calming, stress reduction, recovery, cure, and immune system reinforcement.

And if your kid has a severe problem, there are no contraindications.

Relaxation and sophrology help the child become mindful of its body diagram and manage tension and whether he or she has a phobia (competition, examination, interview, driving license).

Society pressure and overweight

Self-image...

Modern culture returns a body picture that is unreal and stereotypical: It induces shame, permanent unhappiness, and occasionally envy. There are so many negative and damaging feelings over time that take patients through a vicious circle and block any effort in their personal and professional growth.

The food industry stressed eating behavior problems by convenient access to food, whether it be in the community, in the museum, on the highway, at the resort. Thus it is hard to resist: pulse absorption is, therefore, the standard.

But human beings have never felt as hollow, unserviceable to civilization, and need to be filled with something more than ever: self-service food compensates for this badly identified necessity.

... and dietary allergies

Any citizens have placed in motion careful schemes to discourage these temptations and follow rigid regimes: This is recognized as a cognitive limitation. For you, food becomes "healthy" or "evil."

Others, fascinated with good nutrition, try to regulate something, and diet becomes their life's main topic. Thoroughly researched farmers supply them. They extract many foods that are regarded as toxins and are concerned with the consistency and conservation of the materials... Food is medication "I feed healthily, so I'm never going to die." No space for fun or experimentation!

This behavioral condition, which a psychiatrist only diagnoses, is called orthorexia. These individuals are socially excluded, guilty of the minor discrepancy, and, in the worst case, sink into depression. The French population is impaired by 3%.

Release the Feelings

An overweight individual is not a person without a will: The reverse is that it requires a willingness to maintain all these stringent diets, but these can not be used correctly.

Know all about eating habits that trigger this weight disparity.

What feelings or perceptual limits do you have? What makes you hurry to frozen meats and bread after a day's work in the evening? Why do you consume the chocolate bar when you get upset? What do you do... why don't you save too many calories when your body is hungry? What did you do for this body to martyrdom it too much? What do you mean by this?

Welcome the emotions by eating carefully

This technique transforms your dietary patterns and loses weight without depriving you!

- Learn to know who is starving in you?
- Observe the sensations of nature
- Take the opportunity to supply the body with the resources it truly wants.
- Embrace the feelings when they arise

Chapter 2; Physical Hunger

Recognizing Physical Hunger

Phase 1: Assess whether or not the condition necessitates hunger.

Five distinct forms of stimuli activate present overeating programming. The below is a list of both of them:

- Social Incentives: They feed to deal with feelings of inadequacy or to express a shared connection in the hopes of connecting with others. There is scientific proof that when we provide in a group setting, we eat pretty little.
- Sensual Trigger: Pass by the Bakery, Eat Donuts at Work, Advertise Food for Food on TV, or Eat for the opportunity. I didn't have the urge to feed my stomach, but I was unexpectedly hungry after getting the chance to encounter joy. In these situations, the desire to provide is a chance to practice the trained reflex, a pleasurable response to external stimuli. We weren't hungry until we noticed the food on the phone.
- The Motivation for Thought: Eating as a product of a self-condemning cognitive debate. We offend ourselves, and overeating, ironically, typically reprimands us for lack of willpower.
- Physiological Trigger: Whether you eat due to a physical reaction (e.g., headache or other pain).

Eating in reaction to boredom, stress, exhaustion, pain, sadness, rage, anxiety, and loneliness are examples of emotional triggers. These stimuli may be as plain as a loss of body cognition (I need a physical break) or as nuanced as suppressed feelings (I live in a dysfunctional family).

Stage 2: Let Go of The Fascination

My brain is obsessed with food. I'm starving, and my brain is programmed to make me feel obligated to respond to food. This is my new wiring, which makes use of food in reaction to multiple situational stimuli.

Step 3: Identify and address the current requirements.

You have many options on how to best react to the signal, depending on the circumstance.

- Social Trigger: I will try a couple of little bites and rave about the food to appease my need to communicate with others. Much better, you'll be able to launch a lively discussion on something other than food.
- TCB Answer: This isn't a physical hunger pang. This is the drive I have to fit into the culture.
- Sensual Trigger: Remembering my traditional exposure to food's visual appeal. Until I saw the meal, I confess I wasn't hungry. We must acknowledge that this is not physical hunger but rather an automatic reaction to the unexpected.
- TCB Answer: This isn't a physical hunger pang. My Pavlov's reaction to powerfully charged stimuli looks like this. I continue to take pride in the pleasure that food offers. I'll feel better if I eat this good.
- Motivation: Recognize your typical response to depressive emotions, pain, and discomfort. It is a common human reflex to alleviate mental tension. Alternative and meaningful approaches to cope with feelings of inadequacy are available to me.
- TCB Answer: This isn't a physical hunger pang. Eating is a means for me to de-stress and weaken my distressing feelings. I have the skills to live with the painful internal dialogue or get the support I need.

- Physiological Triggers: To help with physical complaints, there are more appropriate resources (medication if needed).
- TCB Answer: This isn't a physical hunger pang. It is a conditioned reaction to body discomfort.
- Mental triggers: You may determine what causes your emotional appetite and take appropriate action.
- TCB Response: This isn't a case of physical starvation. That is my new wiring and average coping strategy.

Step 4: Evaluate The Progress

What happens when you've completed phases 1-3? The scales in the Phase 4-Measures of Improvement and Knowledge of Performance segment will help you chart your progress when implementing new traits. The more you train, the less complicated it would be.

Is it possible for you to react appropriately to each signal? What is your stress level if you replied no? Do you need to de-stress first? What are the best options for meeting the current requirements?

Take the time to prepare a nutritious meal.

Cooking at home has many benefits since it is a means of mindfulness. You choose high-quality, nutrient-dense products on your own. Bear in mind that food retailers prefer low-cost fats and carbs above nutritional sense. You have the discretion of where the calories come from trans fats, added sugars, and so on. They guarantee that no taste enhancers, such as MSG or other brain-disrupting compounds, are available. As previously mentioned, these addictive drugs have the net result of helping you consume more. Creating a nutritious lifestyle is an act of self-love for you and your relatives. It's a marvel of creativity. This thrilling vacation-like activity in Tahiti, Paris, and the Galapagos Islands will save you money. You are free to invest as much time as you wish. To save time in the kitchen, you can use a variety of tips and shortcuts. It's genuine, and it'll help you restore your culinary skills. The master chef inside can be resurrected in only a few hours. I need to get something to eat. Clarify the truth, then go there, park, get some dinner, and eat it there or carry it home. According to the Centers for Disease Control and Prevention (CDC), more than 76 million people get food poisoning per year due to microbes, viruses, and parasites that cause food pollution.

Consider this: you must feed with caution. The consistency of the food you consume is the only aspect that determines 95% of this probability. Is it inexpensive trans-fat oils, a lot of extra sodium, or excess sugar if you don't know who cooks or what recipes they use? What strategies do you use to hold yourself in check?

Taking a Seat in Beauty

If you're eating alone, build an easy and beautiful atmosphere. And if you're starving, getting to an attractive location will take a few minutes. Whether you don't have time, are in a pinch, and choose to feed straight from the freezer, it's a clear indicator that you're typically consumed in foods that trigger anxiety. Although restoring a genetically lean female neural network, this can sound irresistible. This helps to heal the "hungry brain," but it's important to relax before feeding. There are many methods for lowering anxiety levels. Deep breathing, yoga, journaling, active jogging, and everything else appear to work for you to find calm. Always keep track of your success. Are you confident in your ability to set the table? If not, would it be a good idea to figure out what's causing the distress and deal with it?

Eating Adventures

Eating is a secondary practice of a society that promotes multitasking. We should not combine food with our bodies' nutrition. Eating is something we do in the background when performing more essential jobs.

Have you ever switched off the radio in your car while searching for a new address? I intuitively understand that suppressing a speech stimulation enhances the capacity to concentrate on identifying its position. Silence often helps one to focus exclusively on the food and be completely conscious of a meal. You are watching television, using phones, chatting on the internet, reading books, and engaging in other sports are not substitutes for a balanced diet. Mindful meals necessitate undivided focus, which is a perfect way to overeat.

Rewiring will make you remember why you fed for the first time while you were engaged in some operation if you are resistant to silent hoods. It's a tradition that's been passed on for generations. You rarely eat the key attraction.

You can sense internal discussions such as appreciating the food and implicit signals from the body that you are full when you sit calmly and feed. If shutting off opposing stimulation causes panic, take a deep breath and write down the discomfort source.

If you're dining with your mates, ask them to join you in the careful preparation of your meal. It's preferable to toggle off as many obstacles as necessary after your meal than to overeat while multitasking. Talk to the senses and how food tastes to you. Slow food doesn't have to be severe to be successful. It's also a smart thing to tell the family that food isn't a competition. Encourage the family to carefully chew on each food item, inspecting the flavor, smell, and odor. Inquire into their thoughts, praise them for winning brownie points, thank them for their blessings, and encourage their relatives to share their meals.

Often keep track of your progress: After a meal, how do you feel in silence? Are you willing to shut out all noise and feed in peace? Is it easier to eat if you practice this property?

Take pleasure in your meal.

The slim ladies, of course, have an internal conversation of pleasure and appreciation: "This is delicious." It even saturates. Shoveling food not only misses a taste of spice, but it also excludes the entertainment center. Since you're not impressed by it, you'll need more food to meet gourmet merchants.

We agree that the existing tradition of not attending for the sake of dining contributes to this aversion to internal debate. Our conversations are primarily focused on something other than our bodies, but they mainly focus on challenges, worries, and existing to-do lists.

If you pay close attention to what you consume and love it, you will see that the restoration of naturally slender women's wiring is near.

Always keep track of your success. How do you feel now that you've enabled yourself to have an internal debate regarding the enjoyment of eating? If you feel safe having this conversation? If you answered no, what are the challenges you face in achieving this trait?

Small Snacks

You can burn more calories and get the same amount of enjoyment if you overeat food. We would accept that we have previously made many attempts. While we learn to take smaller bites, it is prudent to eat some meals with a small spoon in a wheel's shape. However, once you've made progress in this area, you'll need to increase the scoop size. The reason for this is that if you take a small bite simply because the spoon is empty, the neural network will not be restored, leaving you utterly reliant on the tool.

Put your fork down.

You are advised to feed your heart's content, regardless of where your fork or tableware is put in a bite. We're able to savor every slice, every nuance, every flavor, and every feeling. Eating is a game, not a competition. It's a sensual journey. Arashi thwarts the plan.

Often keep track of your progress: How do you feel after finishing a whole meal and taking a slice with a fork? What is your extent of apprehension? Do you want to savor a delicacy of food?

Chapter 3; Physical Hunger vs. Emotional Hunger

Hunger is a sensation that occurs when an individual has a strong urge to feed. It comes from the hypothalamus and is expressed by liver receptors." This is how Wikipedia defines it. Would this term make us understand what it is to be hungry?

Yeah, however, the mental or sensory dimensions of feeding that we undergo daily are not part of or regarded from a physiological viewpoint. Conscious eating can help us appreciate the many types of hunger we experience.

Is Food Capable of Satisfying Both Types of Hunger?

While the five senses are the most prevalent triggers of hunger, it is necessary to note that other influences may often trigger our hunger patterns.

- Actual Hunger: It refers to the physiological desire in the stomach.

Food prepared with care allows one to understand this fully. Your stomach sounds empty and makes rumbling and gurgling sounds when you're starving. Extreme hunger will make you feel dizzy, irritable, or tired, making it difficult to concentrate. The body must be fed and nurtured in this case.

- Emotional Hunger: You feel happier when you feed.

The need to feel comfortable, to relieve the discomfort, or simply to feel more. When people are sad, angry, or frustrated, they consume chocolates or cookies. Many of us don't eat enough because when we eat without thinking, it explains a sense of pain inside, which can be misinterpreted as actual hunger.

Hunger can also be experienced as an instinct, and it can be far worse than actual need. It is restricted to a particular form of food and exists more in the mouth than in the stomach, and it remains no matter how much vacuum we ingest.

The below are some physical and mental hunger symptoms to look out for.

- Signs of malnutrition are apparent:
- A gurgling throat
- Failure to perform
- Energy scarcity
- Sensation like a gnawing gut
- The success of an empty stomach
- You have a headache.
- Emotional symptoms of hunger:
- Feeding when you're in a poor mood
- Keep track of what you consume, eat less, or deprive yourself of a certain amount of food.
- When you're finished, there's not enough food, and you're starving.
- Walk over to the refrigerator and unlock the handle; ensure that you're there.
- Felt hungry but unable to feed
- You'll never be happy, no matter how much you consume.
- Eating on autopilot
- Eat while you're satisfied and proud of yourself.

It would be easier to lose weight once you understand the distinction between physical and mental hunger. When you hear about the different aspects of need, you'll only consume when you're mentally starving. It's just a suggestion: any time you finish something, take a break and ask yourself, "What hunger do I feel?"

If you're physically starving, you can eat something right away. If not, take the required measures to figure out your emotions and work with them. Take a break if you're sleepy, and then calm down and meditate for 10 minutes if you're stressed or restless.

To reach your weight-loss goal, you'll need the complete help of your conscious and subconscious minds. Otherwise, the transition is not required or lasting, and this is undoubtedly the case when it comes to appetite control.

Allow me to provide you with some background information. Your conscious mind is concerned with your will, while your subconscious mind is involved with your protection, trust, and comfort. If your conscious mind desires one thing and your subconscious mind wants something different, you're going to be frustrated.

So, what would you do if the aware and subconscious minds disagreed?

So, how do you tell if they are?

Okay, since diet is the dilemma you're trying to fix, you'll need a powerful mental resource than food. There are various techniques to choose from, and you should find one that fits you.

EFT is one of my favorite techniques for breaking down interpersonal walls and removing ambiguity from the aware and subconscious mind. When your conscious and subconscious minds find an emotional coping strategy that functions for you, it can put your optimistic weight loss into balance.

If you impose a diet on your mind and body, they will protest and fight back. They oppose a dietary ban, and they want to help you in a dangerous situation and see a diet as a challenge to your health. However, how can you control what you do in your mind and body? Will you depend on willpower to hold your appetite under control? No, not precisely, and not often.

Enable me to demonstrate.

The reality is that naturally, thin people don't have to battle starvation or use it all of the time. We don't feel hungry, which is why it's so interesting that they recognize the feeling as real physical hunger when we begin to encounter the effects of an empty stomach.

However, most people on a weight-loss journey have forgotten this desire, or even their method of eating themselves, since this capacity was never developed in childhood. It's similar to being able to walk normally. If you were limited to a chair as an infant, you might not have acquired the courage to move. The following are confirmed for the bulk of dietitians: • Emotional exhaustion and physical appetite are misunderstood. The diet-induced need has the purpose of teaching the dietitian to ignore the body's hunger signals. If an individual is confined to a chair for long enough, they can lose their ability to move, as in the case above.

- It can make it difficult to know whether you're hungry or whole. Through this simple EFT tapping, you will retrain yourself to recognize whether you are starving or not. When you think you're hungry, tap as seen.
- I let my body and mind guide me, even though I'm not sure if I'm physically or emotionally hungry.

This whole sentence should be tapped on each point. Slowly press on it. It should be tapped. Tell the terms steadily by clicking the keys. We are progressive because Silvia Hartmann's discovery of incremental EFT is an excellent guide and a revelation.

Repeat the process of taping the whole statement on all of the points you usually use for at least 5 minutes. Slow EFT may be replicated with the following information.

Is my stomach empty, or do I need warmth, food, or protection? I trust my body and mind to lead me safely and calmly."

At the very least, give it 5 minutes and then evaluate your output. Get enough to eat if you feel physically starved. Attempt to sit down and chew it gently and intentionally. Relax in the most current culinary experience for your mind and body.

Meanwhile, if you think you are emotionally starving and ask if you have food, remember that a score of ten is abysmal, and a score of zero is acceptable, indicating how bad you would be. If there is worth greater than zero, click it as usual before you have nutritional peace at that point.

Emotional Emptiness as opposed to physical Hunger

Emotional feeding and getting or retaining an abundance of body weight are the most common causes, in my opinion. You used to feed to alleviate mental discomfort in one manner or another, probably in ways you don't even understand.

However, you might argue that I am stressed as a result of my eating habits. You're not content, or at peace, so it worries you. On the other hand, the ability to feed declines after repeatedly releasing suppressed mental tension, often vanishing for an entire day or even longer.

There are two groups of mental overeaters, in my opinion:

- Those who are perplexed and compelled to do it but cannot see how it soothes their feelings.

If you fall into the second group, let me show you something that could be useful. Declare to yourself that you would go a whole day without overeating, and if you have the temptation, deny it entirely. Instead, settle down with a sheet of paper and a pen and jot down any terrible thoughts. After a day, revisit these thoughts. It's the feelings that go into your emotional food!

Then, what precisely is an emotion?

Okay, feelings may be thought of as a warning to the subconscious that something has to be taken care of. For example, when we are near a fire and feel terror, the fear keeps us protected by holding us at a safe distance from the dangerous fire.

It goes away safely until we've completed the necessary analysis to adapt to the feeling and what it teaches us. However, as we relax or divert our mind away from it, the experience returns. Because the cause has not been solved, no diet would again be able to relieve emotional hunger. As a result, you must understand the distinction between eating to ease discomfort and eating to satisfy a physical need.

Using EFT to feed is one way to know whether you're mentally or physically hungry. It's a physical deprivation if you tap for around 10 minutes every day and sound hungry. It was an emotional deprivation as the hunger subsided. Another easy trick is to utilize the way need expresses itself:

- There is an emotional hunger that is both immediate and urgent.

When the food is digested, physical malnutrition becomes more widespread. When you consume nutritious meals, you will notice that your physical appetite begins to develop a few hours after your last meal. For instance, you can approximately predict when you will be ready for lunch a certain amount of hours after breakfast, just as you can expect when you will be prepared for your afternoon snack and dinner. So, how are you going to put this valuable knowledge to use?

The next time you're sleepy, take a minute to relax and observe the sensation. Stand back, relax, and study yourself from inside. Is it easy to arrive to establish an imminent and pressing need, or does it take time to join and increase awareness? Have the courage to sit with it, calm your mind, and observe the sensation if you are suddenly and urgently starving.

How does it make you feel?

Was it a burning need to experience something in your gut, a deep boulder in your throat, or something else entirely?

- Where does the sensation, the texture, or the color come from? Is it simply tension that you're experiencing?

What does it entail for you?

You should only use EFT if you come up with a tapering emotion. If you need to feel something in your mouth, for example, tap "As if I have to feel something in my mouth..."

Chapter 4; Eating Disorders

Binge Eating

Food may become a source of anxiety. It's difficult to say how badly you like it. Why does eating a loaf of bread taste so good? The sense of relaxation that comes with carrying a whole gallon of ice cream and consuming it with a spoon is comparable to the warmth that a heated blanket will provide. Binge eating is described as eating an excessive amount of food over an extended period. People often gorge on unhealthy items at first, although those in rehab can notice that they binge on "healthy" foods such as fruits, tea, and water. It's a habit of overeating to the point that you feel physically and emotionally sick. These times are typically spent isolated, and there is often a sense of guilt and humiliation involved.

Binging isn't fun, or at least not all of the time. At first, there's the enjoyment of flavor and texture, as well as the comfort of just how much food you're eating. After the fourth or fifth sandwich, taco, or slice of pie, it begins to dawn on you that you shouldn't be doing this and that you should quit at any point. Yet we continue to feed, trying to drown out the rational voice in our minds.

According to estimates, binge eating disorder impacts 3 to 5% of women and 2% of adults. However, because of the shame associated with eating disorders, even other people go undiagnosed. Those who have never experienced an eating problem may still have a rough time knowing it. People can notice that you are doing anything dangerous if you have bulimia, which is when they become concerned. Repeated vomiting will harm your body on the inside, damaging your throat and liver. Anorexia and binge feeding are both harmful, but they aren't often seen as such, mainly whether you are overweight or underweight. Many that binge feed while being skinny doesn't seem to have a problem. Some people might also say things like, "You can put on some weight," or "You're all skin and bones!" It also applies to people who are obese or anorexic. People aren't likely to be as worried if you're 275 pounds and go through times of deprivation. Some people may also promote it. Those figures represent almost one out of every 20 individuals you will encounter, and there are also too many contradictory philosophies about binge feeding, overeating, anorexia, and bulimia.

Many binge eating disorders may experience anorexia or bulimia due to their binge cycles or have had them before the binge. Both are highly dangerous, which may contribute to individual suffering in humiliation and agony, which just helps to intensify their illness. We do unhealthy stuff and then attempt to make amends by doing things we believe are reasonable. However, there are all bad habits. Anorexics and bulimics do this because they feel it is healthier for their bodies to solve the overeating they placed their bodies through first. However, it's yet another dysfunctional coping strategy.

Bulimia

Binge-feeding episodes typically follow bulimia, but specific individuals can experience bulimia after developing a binge eating disorder. The bulk of diagnostics include patients who gorge on food in amounts that are much greater than what an average individual can drink. Bulimia is a reaction to a binge, and it typically includes individuals purging themselves of the food they already consumed.

Bulimia is more than mere vomiting. Many individuals would acquire laxatives to consume them directly after a binge to help pass things into their bodies fast enough to prevent adding weight. Bulimia may allow you to lose weight, but it is a harmful habit that will kill several other aspects of the body in the process. To begin with, it places a great deal of strain on the body and mind. Bulimics are also passive sufferers who maintain their acts secret from others.

It may also be incredibly detrimental to the heart. Since our hearts weren't made to take in needless laxatives or the discomfort of vomiting up daily, certain bulimics will have a heart attack, mainly though they are dangerously underweight. It may also induce gastrointestinal and digestive disorders, including inflammation, gastric reflux, and gastroparesis, a disease in which the stomach muscles are partly paralyzed.

Some may assume you're doing it for the publicity. When I was throwing up, I knew people who claimed their parents or siblings told them they only needed promotion, particularly those who weren't underweight. People may assume you can't be bulimic if you're not a size 0 with transparent bone shadows or a gaunt-looking face. This illness isn't an excuse to draw publicity to itself.

Excuses have been commonplace. Many that compete in physical events will have the most reasons. Wrestlers who are struggling to make weight will probably claim that they are doing so to pass the time before weigh-in. Participants in beauty pageants and brides-to-be will say that they are just doing so to step into an outfit. People will say they're specifically aiming to drop twenty pounds before giving up. They are indeed justifications, and many bulimics have created them too.

There is a great deal of guilt inherent in the procedure. Bulimia is typically the product of a psychiatric disorder like anxiety or depression. If there isn't one at all, one would most definitely appear. It's a method of concealing the binge cycle and then the purge period. Though there is fear to purge shortly after binging, these often have to be different events. You could binge feed in your car during your lunch break at work and then run to the bathroom until your body begins to absorb the food properly. A coworker could pause and talk on the drive to work, but your heart will be pounding the whole time, praying you'll make it to the toilet in time to throw up your big lunch.

Anorexia nervosa is a disorder in which

Males account for 25% of anorexia patients. They also have a greater prevalence of more severe related health complications since they don't mention their illnesses — males are thought to be immune to anorexia. We place too much focus on avoiding being "big," or overweight and obese; in our culture, we often ignore the risks of being underweight. Self-image is so twisted that we'll starve ourselves and force our bodies to vomit only to fit into an idealized image of what the perfect body should be.

Anorexia is defined by an extreme reduction in food consumption, to the extent that you might not be feeding at all. Anorexics have skewed body perceptions and a deep apprehension of adding weight. They usually consume less than one meal a day, and their snacks are generally smaller than other people's. Anorexics may begin to expel their bodies, but they're usually is not much to purge in the first place.

Excessive Intake

Unhealthy eating patterns such as malnutrition times, vomiting, laxative misuse, and crash dieting have also been recorded by approximately 35% of girls. That's a startlingly fast pace. That suggests that out of every three people you meet, at least one has subjected her body to an unnatural procedure in the name of improving her body image.

Overeating isn't good for you, but it's not as bad as binge-feeding. The majority of people you meet have overeaten at least once in their lives. Who hasn't overindulged at a Thanksgiving buffet, a Vegas buffet, or even a weekend pizza party? Overeating occurs when you don't listen to your body when it tells you it's finished or when you try to take advantage of the plenty of food available. Overeating isn't going to damage you, mainly if it's an accidental event. When it happens daily, it may become an issue.

Why Can People Overeat?

Since women's general view of eating disorders is that they aspire to be slim and lose weight, the underlying emotional causes are often ignored. When you think about bulimia, you probably think of a cheerleader who wants to lose weight, but you probably don't think of a solid male wrestler who wants to lose weight. When you hear about anorexia, the thinnest individual you meet comes to mind, not the biggest. Although eating disorders can have clinical signs that show themselves outward over time, we can't always conclude that anyone who appears a certain way isn't suffering from a binge eating disorder.

If we were to remove the stigmas, we would have better instruction, which would aid preventive initiatives. It's humiliating to admit that you have a hunger addiction when everybody feeds! Not everybody consumes alcohol, even those who do will be able to agree that they can see how it may become a concern. It's humiliating and disgusting to say you've consumed ten McDonald's Double Cheeseburgers, but it's challenging to come out — except though you're desperate for support.

Eight out of ten women would confess to attending a significant occurrence in their lives because they were disappointed with their appearance. We are more concerned about whether or not anyone seems to be "fat" than about whether or not they are throwing up in the shower. We are sometimes oblivious to how they speak to someone, and we don't know that some of the things we say may be triggering.

Any people suffer from deep-seated anxiety issues. Others have stumbled into it and have no idea what they are doing. Whatever began it, it must be halted, and we'll spend the rest of the book guides you through your rehabilitation.

Bad Eating Habits

Emotional eating involves consuming vast volumes of calories, mainly junk snacks, to alleviate tension. Emotions are blamed for around 75% of overeating. All of us feel that feeding would provide us with immediate relief from our mental pain.

As a consequence, most of us begin to use diet as a tension reliever. Isolation, anger, boredom, sadness, anxiety, and tension, as well as some kind of mental issue affecting interpersonal relationships and poor self-esteem, both lead to eating disorders and weight gain.

About what triggers eating disorders is the first and only approach to avoid eating disorders. Suppose you realize why you'll quickly discover healthier strategies to cope with your anxiety problems and maintain your eating patterns.

What Are Stimuli and How Can You Know Them?

Emotions and eating disorders are classified into five categories:

- Emotional: consuming food to alleviate boredom, fear, fatigue, weakness, anger, sadness, or loneliness.
- Physiological: Physical stimuli often drive excessive eating. You can experience discomfort as a result of missed meals, managing headaches, or experiencing pain.
- Situation: You might be overeating when you have the opportunity to consume. Going to the cinema, viewing TV, and other activities are also examples of eating.
- Physical: Eating, assisting someone, or becoming self-conscious in social situations.

- Thoughts: Indulging in excessive eating as a means of self-punishment or low self-worth.

How Can You Get Out of That Bad Habit?

The first move is to find out what triggers you to overeat. However, this would not help you change your dietary behaviors on its own. You'll have to interrupt poor eating behaviors that have formed due to social discomfort or unpleasant conditions.

You'll need alternatives to diet to achieve this. If you're hungry, you'd instead do something else, or read a book or magazine, do deep breathing exercises, go for a long walk or jog, chat to a mate, play games, or do housework.

Sometimes, simple distractions are insufficient. If you notice that the options you've tried aren't effective, you may need to consider a more aggressive solution like yoga, calming techniques, hypnotherapy, or counseling. These methods help you identify stress problems and teach you how to cope positively and effectively.

Reward yourself with a massage or other self-loving practice as you successfully incorporate coping strategies in your eating disorders, helping you accomplish your targets.

Here are a few weight-loss ideas that will help you feel at home in your new gown!

Overweight is the century's challenge, and nearly anyone we know tries to keep or lose weight. This method may be one of the most challenging trials ever, with significant implications for the individual's existence.

To lose weight safely and efficiently, there are specific guidelines to obey. One would be able to recognize whey as the cause of their obesity. Is it a nagging injury, a sluggish schedule, or a drained mind?

If somebody doesn't grasp the underlying cause, they won't be able to lose weight quickly. However, due to certain emotional factors, a specific technique must be utilized. One can lose weight fast with the correct attitude and determination.

Any dietitian would propose a weight-loss regimen that involved consuming healthy meals six days a day, consuming lots of water and fiber, and keeping to a weekly workout schedule.

In comparison, small life-changing strategies may be applied easily. However, if an individual is experiencing mental distress, a weight reduction strategy like this would be of little use. If you're nervous, you separate yourself, and your metabolism slows down.

Many individuals are in a state of internal distress and frustration due to their failure to lose weight after a weight-loss regimen. As a result, getting to the root of the stress-inducing issue is critical.

Many citizens are now irritated for various causes. As a consequence, qualified physicists are now delivering innovative stress-reduction approaches all over the world. When a psychiatrist uses the Emotional Liberty Tactic (EFT), he or she may relieve frustration.

To achieve outstanding performance, EFT needs a variety of processes and methods. For weight loss, EFT includes tapping, which is a form of acupuncture that induces pressure points.

Tapping for weight reduction is fast gaining popularity because it is easy to do and has no harmful consequences. Someone should obtain medical care before embarking on a weight-loss regimen. As a result, both of these factors are highly beneficial to the client and will most certainly support anyone dealing with such a challenge.

If you eat while you're bored, depressed, or anxious, emotional binge feeding is a problem. What is the significance of binge eating? The most crucial factor in stopping emotional eating is because it contributes to weight gain over time.

A binge will continue for many hours, days, weeks, or even months. Binge eating is not recommended for someone who has gained weight and is attempting to retain their current weight or for someone who is consciously working to reduce weight. This chapter will assist you in ending your consuming binge.

If you want to stop binge feeding, the first thing you can do is get rid of unnecessary fast food from your house. Remember that you won't be tempted to consume those fatty snack snacks if you don't have them on hand, so stock your kitchen with balanced, fresh foods, including fruits and vegetables.

However, if you're stressed and searching for a way to get rid of it by binge feeding, follow a well-balanced diet and stop carrying more weight.

Putting all calories in and out of reach is another method to avoid emotional feeding. The more food you see, the more hungry you can get. The majority of people binge feed, and they don't pay attention, and even that, they're starving.

Many people who like getting a bag of chips on their laps or nearby when eating will soon note that the bag is empty. The straightforward reason is that the tv show attracted their focus, so if mental eating is to be stopped, all foods must be held out of sight.

More water is an effective way to prevent emotional feeding. It is important to consume 8-12 glasses of water a day. According to doctors, consuming ten water drinks a day can help you fill your stomach and cope with fake hunger, leading to binge feeding.

You don't have to drink all 8-12 glasses at once; spread them out during the day. Between and after meals, drink more water. One point to keep in mind is that you cannot substitute soda for water; water must be sweet. Instead of soda, drink tea.

Binge eating is fuelled by boredom or depression.

If you're bored and sound starving (fake hunger), my suggestion is to find something to occupy your time, and the false need will disappear before you know it, saving you from binge feeding. Go out with a friend, play games, or read a book; get occupied, and the false hunger can vanish.

Consider something better and more accessible than food to help with the suffering, whether you're sad or mentally disturbed. You should also see a psychologist to identify the main problem and formulate a strategy for resolving it.

If you binge feed while you're stressed or emotionally upset, you're setting yourself up for a habit that may be much riskier than you realize. Don't be one of the individuals that promise themselves, "I'll stop binge feeding because I'm no longer depressed or irritated," when they're binge eating.

Binge-eaters are all that neglect self-control — do you have to be one of them? Know that only you and you alone can say you to feed, and only you and you alone can save yourself from overeating. If you're serious about losing weight, you'll need to maintain a healthy outlook and the determination to resist binge feeding.

Emotional feeding is the most effective way to sabotage every flat stomach diet to prevent you from reaching your weight reduction targets. These four ideas will help you avoid self-sabotage and keep on board with your diet schedule.

Brushing your teeth is the simplest way to stop emotional feeding. Brushing your teeth after a meal is suitable for your dental health, but who wants to damage their freshly brushed teeth, particularly when they're flavored with dark chocolate and spearmint?

Hold the weight reduction targets in mind the next time you reach into the candy dish. Mind that you're working and what you're looking towards. Why don't you try slipping into a pair of jeans? Lose 10 pounds or just be more at home in shorts?

Whatever the weight-loss ambitions are, sugar won't help you reach them, and it can just make things more complicated. It would be much simpler to dig into those goodies if you remember your goals.

Try writing down your feelings instead of eating them.

Take a piece of paper or a notebook to write down your views on these delectable treats.

Not only can writing down your feelings and feelings help you get over the extreme candy cravings, but it can also help you spot some changes or inconsistencies in your behavior.

Finally, and maybe most importantly, drinking water will help you curb your sweet cravings. We don't consume nearly enough water, and we misunderstand our sugar cravings because we're thirsty. Water will not only quench your hunger, but it will also fill you up, leaving no space for dessert!

When we're at our most vulnerable, mental eating comes to the fore. However, remembering these techniques any time you take a sugar pill will help you reach your weight reduction targets much faster.

Good Eating Habits

You may be wondering what the first step is to interrupt the cycle of destructive eating patterns that lead to your mood problems and making you feel exhausted all of the time. Accepting that the issue is when it all begins is the solution to specific questions. But there's more to it than that.

Begin with a nutritious and well-balanced meal.

When you skip meals, you're more likely to binge in the middle of the day, resulting in a calorie and sugar overdose. One-third of Americans became obese as a result of this. Let's not forget the effect that breakfast has on your energy levels as well as those pounds you're striving to shed, so your metabolism slows down drastically.

What you crave is what you drink a lot of: When you consume more food, you can desire more sugar, as well as more vegetables and protein. Discipline is essential for cultivating healthy eating behaviors that can become second nature. The long-term results would significantly exceed the happy shifts in brain chemistry that come from bad eating habits.

Drinking more water if you're starving can help you stop cravings: People aren't allowed to consume soda or fake juices, and if you believe this is a safe and hydrating activity, think differently. It's because we buy all of the so-called "hydration" publicity hype that informs us we're taking care of our bodies when, in fact, it's just another part of our overall healthy eating and drinking behaviors. Consider drinking more water as fuel for your attempts to burn weight, maintain your skin looking great, and boost your cells' ability to function correctly.

Your blood sugar would be controlled if you eat balanced 5 hours a day: Do you know the most popular explanation for people struggling to consume more than 2-3 meals a day? It's a day, as you're well aware. Why do you like to know when I'll be able to consume five or even six meals a day? To start, you must recognize that an authentic meal will vary from a blueberry muffin and an apple to a handful of almonds with a banana to a hard-boiled egg with a fruit/veggie smoothie. Change your mind on how a meal can fill your plate to include all big food groups. It would have an immediate impact on your overeating behaviors, making a significant improvement to your blood sugar and energy levels. Even as in anything, the beginning can be difficult, but it is well worth it.

Interrupt the mental feeding loop by doing the following: Start a diary that contains your regular eating patterns and give you a simple view of how things are progressing, or pick up a new hobby to draw your focus away from food. It's wildly successful in the evenings (when the cravings for junk food are high). The most crucial thing is not to hesitate to set yourself up for success; as previously said, this involves preparation and much-needed discipline.

No more excuses, no more telling yourself that if you indulge a bit, you'll feel happier in the long run. Instead, consider the long-term advantages of this move, as well as the sense of satisfaction and trust you'll gain once you start to see the results you desire in your life. Remember that being good does not imply going hungry; it just means eating various nutritious foods.

The reality regarding most diets is that they all struggle at some stage. If you're tired of crash diets and work to find out how to gain strength and shed weight that won't go anywhere, you can begin by retraining yourself to eat properly. When it comes to shedding the last few stubborn pounds and revealing the muscles you worked so hard for, a few minor improvements in your regular eating patterns will make a huge difference.

Your environment, diet, and dietary behaviors all play a role in the physical well-being and the results you see in the mirror. Physical activity and good nutritional behaviors are the most critical factors in achieving and sustaining a balanced weight and lean muscle mass. When you go food shopping or are considering what to do for dinner, break away from your everyday schedule. Please give it a goal to consume an extensive range of healthy foods from all food classes. Instead of what you're eating now, switch to high-fiber whole grains, restrict saturated fat consumption, and switch to low-fat dairy goods. Get in the habit of checking diet labels and ingredients, and you'll have more say over what you eat.

Aside from bettering your dietary patterns, you can implement a workout regimen that focuses on meeting your weight-loss and muscle-building objectives. Start with a pair of dumbbells or a few simple exercises like squatting and pushups, and build your way up to utilizing your body weight. When you're just starting, don't go more than three days a week, so your muscles need time to heal and expand in workouts. When you've gotten used to a schedule, continue to alternate muscle groups any time so that each group has time to heal. For most beginners, three sets of each weight are recommended, with no more than 10 to 12 reps per pair. If you find that 12 brokers are too easy, you can progress to the next stage.

Don't get discouraged if you add a little weight at the beginning of your trip. Note, you're adding muscle and losing weight, so if the numbers on the scale increase, that could be the product of your new development. It would be beneficial to miss the stages for a short time and then focus solely on measurements. That will save you from succumbing to the desire to go on a hunger diet, which will just slow down your metabolism if the numbers on the scale don't seem to be going.

Water also plays a part in the processes that contribute to the development of muscles. Water consumption, regular activity, and a balanced diet are the most critical factors in achieving and maintaining the muscle-building and weight-loss targets. Some people find it immensely useful to participate with a weight loss partner or someone who will keep you motivated and give you the little boost you need to keep going.

Nutritional Habits That Are Good For You

The majority of us live busy, hectic lives and aspire to fulfill our hopes and aspirations. With excessive pressures and a heavy workload, most of us lack our dietary consumption and the kinds of food we consume regularly. We develop poor eating behaviors as a result. Any of us may eat inappropriately without realizing it, depending on the eating patterns our parents instilled in us as children. The real trick to smart eating is to develop successful behaviors.

What does it entail to have good eating habits? Is that carbon dioxide? What's the case with protein? What are fats? — What are such phytochemicals? What are those antioxidants? How much of each nutrient can we consume? The volume of information available on the internet and in the physical world, such as magazine magazines, is enough to leave most of us nostalgic and perplexed. It doesn't have to be challenging to eat well. For the most part, we live entire and chaotic lives, but straightforward and easy-to-follow ideas are what we seek. Here are 12 easy-to-follow ideas to help you start nurturing and integrate them into your regular meal schedule.

- **Tip #1: Take a morning multivitamin every day.**

Just one multivitamin tablet a day is needed. A regular multivitamin can fill up the holes in your diet enough to make a difference since most people lack one or two micronutrients.

- **Tip #2: Drink two glasses of water before each dinner.**

It will not only hold you hydrated, but it will also cause you to consume less. This can help you feel less hungry, allowing you to consume less, stop you from overeating at each meal, and help you lose weight.

- **Tip # 3: Start your day with heavy meals and steadily reduce your parts.**

Start the day with breakfast as the main meal, steadily increasing the volume of food consumed as the day progresses. Our metabolism is fastest at the start of each day, but it decreases dramatically as the day progresses. Having big meals late at night is terrible for your well-being and can encourage you to add weight excessively.

- **Tip #4: Eat nutritious foods at the appropriate times.**

Complex carbohydrates make up 50-60% of the diet. This is since complex carbs take a long time for the body to absorb, supplying nutrition during the day without triggering insulin spikes, contributing to fat accumulation. However, it's advised that you have a meal high in essential carbohydrates after your exercise to replenish your glycogen supplies, which are your fat reserves that were depleted throughout your workout. The key is to eat the best food at the right moment.

- **Suggestion #5: Feed regularly during the day.**

Every 2-3 hours, eat something. This will improve your metabolism and enable your body to lose fat more effectively. You'd probably be less sluggish, and you'd be getting endless calories from the food you consume all day.

- **Tip #6: Feed wisely.**

Stuff that seems to be greasy would have given you a heads-up that it includes harmful fats. This is something that common sense will warn you not to do.

- **Take a rest.**

We all have those meals that we like eating. Do not transform them into forbidden pleasures. I don't consume them regularly. Consider how many you eat of them and how much you can cut down on if your well-being is at risk. One method is to change your preferred meals during the week, allowing them once or twice a week. If you're having difficulty avoiding hunger, consider consuming your favorite meal in smaller amounts throughout the day rather than in the evening.

- **Tip #8: Make a cup of tea.**

Incorporate orange, black, or white tea into the everyday routine. Tea has been shown in studies to supply the body with antioxidants essential in combating severe diseases, including heart disease and cancer. Apart from that, these teas are abundant in antioxidants and anti-aging agents, which may reduce wrinkles.

- **Tip # 9: Arrange all of the onions in a pile.**

Onions are a great source of heart-healthy flavonoids. Furthermore, they are an outstanding source of antioxidants.

- **Tip # ten: Have tomatoes in your diet.**

Using a lot of tomato-based items will help reduce the cancer risk. This is because they're high in lycopene, a carotenoid that's thought to lower cancer risk. According to research, men who eat several tomatoes have a reduced chance of getting prostate cancer.

- **Tip # 11: Still feed with your skin on.**

Leave the skin on fruits and vegetables, such as potatoes, after consuming them. To remove the skin, you'll be tossing away the heavy-duty fiber and nutrients. However, that does not imply that the skin on meat items such as chicken should be left on, which is harmful and high in cholesterol.

Chapter 5; Power of Meditation

What is the concept of meditation?

Meditation is derived from the Latin term "medicine," which initially meant "natural medicine." Meditation entails separating ourselves from our feelings, voices, and impulses in our minds and observing them independently without making critical or constructive decisions. This method can be used when sweeping, and we don't need to be in a particular position to meditate. We may assume we are contemplating if we do anything from the core. Meditation is the process of concentrating all of one's energy on a particular object.

Meditation is a specific condition of consciousness that can't be forced or generated through willpower. It's close to sleep in this way, so the more we want to sleep, the more aware we'll be. Meditation is a state of mind where the body is deliberately carefree and comfortable, and our soul is released from inner tension and focus. Meditation is more than just sitting or lying down in quiet for five to ten minutes. Meditation does necessitate mindful action. The mind has to stay calm and balanced. Around the exact moment, the brain must remain vigilant to prevent any unwanted ideas or impulses from entering. With our effort, we begin meditation. When we look further within ourselves, though, we see that it is not ourselves that encourages one to reach a state of meditation. Through our conscious focus and authorization, the Supreme or Creator meditates inside and through us.

The aim is to achieve happiness and be rid of intrusive thoughts. In such situations, the meditator experiences a release from the world, and the phenomenon may also be classified as a modified state of consciousness from a psychological standpoint. When we can relax and quiet our hearts, we will experience a new life that has awoken within us. Our internal presence will call upon divine grace, illumination, and forgiveness to flood through and fill this vessel if our mind is discharged and tranquil, and our whole becoming an empty vessel. This occurs while you're meditating.

Meditation's Influence

Because of its various advantages, meditation has been adopted in several traditions for thousands of years: It relieves tension and makes people comfortable. Meditation has primarily psychological effects in the short term, but it still has physical benefits in the long run. Many who practice meditation will gain immediate benefits such as improved balance, calm, and energy, as well as a diminished need for sleep. Physical benefits will be felt after a few months, including returning to natural blood pressure and improved digestion. As a consequence, you can see how valuable it can be in the long term.

For years, the University of California's Neuroscience Laboratory has researched the influence of meditation on the brain's structure. Their most recent analysis contrasted the long-term impact of regular meditators to non-meditators in the brains of regular meditators. According to their observations, long-term meditators' prefrontal cortex is more pronounced than non-meditators, suggesting better cognitive performance. The journal Frontiers of Human Neuroscience reported findings that became a scientific breakthrough since it has long been assumed that brain mass peaks in the early twenties and then gradually narrows (Bae, Hur, Hwang, Jung, Kang, Kim, Kwak, Kwon, Lee, Lim, Cho, & Park, 2019). It was commonly accepted that there was no way to avoid the process. However, it is now understood that the brain maintains certain plasticity and can alter biologically due to meditation. According to previous research, long-term meditators' gray and white matter in the brain also risen in weight. (The former includes brain cells called nerve cells, while the latter contains neuronal cell projections.)

Through maturity, the number of neurons in the cortex varies relatively little. The present sample featured 28 men and 22 women, all of whom were 51 years old and had been meditating for an average of 20 years. The oldest person was 71 years old, and the most seasoned meditator had been doing so regularly for 46 years. The researchers contrasted the patients' brain scans to those of 50 non-meditating members of the control community.

Meditation's benefits may be amplified with regular exercise. According to studies, the more people practiced deep breathing and other meditation exercises, the minor discomfort they had, the stronger their immune systems became, the higher their cortisol levels were, and the lower their blood pressure was. According to the researchers, this illustrates how a person's emotional status will affect his physical health and provides more evidence for why meditation and mantra practice is considered beneficial in Tibetan, Indian, and Ayurvedic medicine.

Hundreds of clinical studies back up meditation's positive therapeutic and fitness effects. Here are a few examples.

The first twenty minutes of meditation trigger a sixteen percent reduction in metabolism. During transcendental meditation, the body relaxes profoundly due to reduced cellular oxygen consumption due to slowed metabolism. It also lowers blood pressure and improves breathing (Dillbeck & Orne-Johnson, 1987). Furthermore, blood pressure drops, and muscle stress and fear fade away as a result. Meditation has been shown to help people overcome persistent distress and boost their self-esteem (Eppley, Abrams, & Shear, 1989). Meditation may also help you calm and de-stress by reducing physiological arousal. A reduction in respiratory rate, oxygen intake, and carbon dioxide exhalation is the syndrome's essence. Breathing becomes rarer and more profound; critical power rises from 450-550 ml at rest to 800-1300 ml (up to 2000 ml for certain master meditators) and stays constant throughout. However, deeper breathing does not compensate for a lower respiratory rate, resulting in a 20% decrease in respiratory volume at rest.

Several sports psychologists agree that meditation may help athletes enhance their performance (Syer, & Conolly, 1984). Meditation can help athletes cope with the intensity of competition, but they can also learn to calm specific muscle groups and sense subtle muscle tension changes with more experience.

The athlete will predict the next event (such as skiing downhill) in such detail through meditation that the activity's visualization is almost completely aligned with the action itself. The skier visualizes himself beginning from the starting spot, gliding down and speeding, avoiding the gates, and completing the race in his mind. An athlete will try to program their muscles and body for optimal outcomes by framing sound output photos.

Meditation's Impact

Since we equate feelings from the depths of the soul with conscious thinking, meditation has tremendous strength. In meditation, the entity is taken through the same frequency as the Inner Self's root, which is the World itself and is thereby directly linked to the Universe's consciousness sphere. Since there is no time limit in this state, the visualized delivery will stretch to the actual level right away. We enjoy various physical and emotional advantages as a consequence of daily meditation. We would feel happier, and concentrating on our breathing reduces our blood pressure and slows our pulse rate, rendering us calmer. It allows us to have a clearer mind, organize our thoughts and feelings, and communicate more effectively at work and in social situations. We can concentrate more quickly and become less overwhelmed as a result. We become more mindful of our feelings, helping us to control them properly. In parts of our lives where we are trapped, we pursue away faster. It aids in the resolution of emotional issues. It aids in the attainment of unity and harmony. We gain a better understanding of ourselves, our surroundings, our lives, and our task. We become optimistic, joyful, and desirable as we embrace ourselves as we are. If we are still in a partnership, this will make it more personal, so the desired spouse will enter our lives if we are single.

What is the concept of directed meditation?

Unlike conventional meditation, directed meditation has a particular target in mind, and it is one of the easiest ways to continue this activity for beginners. It's often referred to as directed visualization. You create imaginary pictures of environments or scenarios where you can recover in this form of meditation. Much of the time, this is done with an instructor's assistance or a mentor who is not often present in the meditation area. Listening to a recording and meditating on it is sufficient.

Not all directed meditations are created equal: It depends on what you intend to do through this exercise. Will you simply want to unwind? How can you get rid of insomnia? Boost your resiliency? Accept a significant change? If you're going to lose weight?

It's necessary to use as many senses as possible during most supervised meditations: The smells, the lights, the voices, and the textures all contribute to the overall experience. Typically, led meditations include music playing in the background to help the mind and body relax: Rain, rainforest, sea waves, or the roar of a waterfall are examples of natural noises, as well as more traditional music such as Native American flutes, tubes, and rattles. Choose your musical background; the main thing is to relax in the best way possible. You can start by doing a short directed meditation for beginners. The fundamental idea is to pay attention to what you're doing and note it in the lesson. Lock your eyes and inhale through your nose and exhale through your mouth for three deep breaths.

Technique of Meditation

Meditation of Consciousness

It's quick to get wrapped up in a cycle of swirling thoughts — worrying about a laundry list of stuff to do, ruminating about past incidents, or contemplating hypothetical potential scenarios — and practicing mindfulness can help. But, precisely, what is attention? It's a behavioral condition that necessitates being wholly immersed in "the moment" so that you can recognize and acknowledge your emotions, feelings, and sensations without judgment.

Mindfulness meditation is a form of mental preparation that enables you to quiet down rushing thoughts, let go of frustration, and relax your mind and body. Mindfulness strategies differ, but most mindfulness meditations contain breathing exercises, internal visualization, body and mind consciousness, and muscle and organ stimulation. Meditation with mindfulness should not involve any props or training (no need for candles, essential oils, or mantras, unless you enjoy it). What you'll need is a cozy seat, three to five minutes of free time, and a judgment-free mindset.

Mindfulness meditation is a technique for becoming genuinely conscious of your emotions. Being aware of where we are and what we do and not being too open about what is going on around us is part of knowledge.

Reflective therapy can be done everywhere. Some people like to unwind in a peaceful environment, shut their eyes, and concentrate on their breathing. You may opt to be awake at any time of day, including commuting to work or performing chores.

When doing mindfulness therapy, you keep track of your emotions and emotions so don't judge them.

- Transcendental meditation: This is an effective practice in which an independently specified rhythm, such as an expression, tone, or short sentence, is replicated in a specific manner. It is performed for 20 minutes twice a day when sitting comfortably next to the eyes.

It is anticipated that by utilizing this method, you would be able to slip into a deep state of relaxation and find inner harmony without needing to pay attention or expend effort.

- Focused Meditation: Directed meditation, also known as guided imagery or simulation, is a form of meditation where you construct relaxing mental images or scenarios.

Guided meditation is one of the most common types of meditation, with millions of people practicing it every day. We'll look at directed meditation and how to perform it in this article.

In its purest form, Driven meditation is a meditation method in which the subject is guided in every phase of his daily practice. From the first step of sitting in a meditative posture to the final process of finishing the meditation, somebody shows you. During meditation, an instructor or coach gives step-by-step instructions for how to meditate. It's an old way of providing students with meditation instructions. This approach was once used to practice meditation in a community environment. Thanks to technological advancement, we no longer need a guru's physical appearance to guide us in meditation. We should perform our meditation practice when listening to a master's direct instruction on pre-recorded CDs or DVDs. If you don't have any meditation master professional CDs or DVDs, you can record yourself reading directed meditation instructions from a book and then play them again.

Furthermore, if a person does not have access to a voice recorder or a DVD player, they can ask friends or relatives to read the written meditation directions aloud during a session. This way, we will reap the benefits of directed meditation without relying on technology.

However, I continue to agree that directed meditation using a pre-recorded CD or DVD is the safest method since it eliminates the need for anyone to be physically present with you to interpret the notes. It also allows you to meditate in a controlled manner even though you're home.

Depending on the techniques the instructor utilizes, directed mediation instructions may take several different types. Vipassana — which includes imagery of the breathing cycle, visual imagining, mantra recitation, a meditation on dancing, a meditation on prayer, and a meditation on mindfulness, among other things — is one of the most popular meditation exercises used in directed meditation. Listening to a master's live instruction is the most convenient way to utilize direct mediation. If this is not practical, the next best choice is to capture the written mediation notes in your voice and then listen to them during your meditation session.

A guide or teacher usually guides this step and thus is "led." To evoke calmness in your calming zone, it is also advised that you use as many senses as possible, such as smell, vibrations, and textures.

- Vipassana Meditation: Vipassana meditation is a traditional Indian meditation method that entails seeing things as they are. It was first taught in India about 2,500 years ago. In the United States, this exercise gave rise to the conscious mediation trend.

Vipassana meditation aims to attain self-transformation by self-examination. This is achieved by paying close attention to the body's sensations to establish a strong bond between the mind and the body. The satisfied account is filled with affection and sympathy as a consequence of the sustained interconnectedness.

In this practice, Vipassana is usually taught throughout a 10-day course. Participants are required to adhere to a series of laws at all times, including abstaining from all intoxicants, lying, stealing, sexual intercourse, and sacrificing any livestock.

- Metta meditation (loving-kindness meditation): Metta meditation, also known as loving-kindness meditation, is the art of directing positive thoughts for others. Hot emotions would be evoked by those who practice reciting related terms and phrases. This can also be observed in mindfulness and vipassana meditation.

It's typically achieved when sitting in a comfortable, relaxing place. You gently and gradually repeat the following phrases after a few deep breaths. "Allow me to be content. I'll be perfect. Enable me to be free. Could I feel at peace and calm?" After a moment of directing this loving-kindness toward yourself, imagine a family member or acquaintance who has helped you and reiterate the mantra, substituting "you" for "I." If you begin to meditate, other members of your family, colleagues, neighbors, or individuals in your life might come to mind. Individuals who are experiencing difficulties with them are often advised to be seen by practitioners.

- Eventually, as a Chakra meditation, you conclude the reflection with the traditional mantra: "Let every being be satisfied everywhere."

Chakra is an ancient Sanskrit word that means "cycle" and can be traced back to India. The chakras relate to the body's energies and spiritual power centers. There would be seven chakras, according to popular belief. Each chakra is located in a separate section of the body and has a distinct hue.

Chakra mediation is a collection of calming exercises aimed at restoring chakra equilibrium and well-being. These methods will display the visual image of any chakra in the body and the related light. Some people like to light incense or use color-coded crystals for each Chakra to concentrate during meditation.

- Yoga meditation: Yoga meditation has its origins in ancient India. Yoga lessons and types differ, but both involve a set of postures and coordinated breathing techniques intended to improve stability and relieve the mind.

The poses necessitate balance and focus, and practitioners are advised to focus less on outside distractions and more on the present moment.

Several considerations affect which mediation style you want to pursue. Tell your doctor which technique will be best for you if you have a health condition and are new to yoga.

Chapter 6; Meditation and Weight Loss

Weight Reduction and Transcendental Therapy

Meditation is commonly used to relax the mind, just as a back massage with the physical body. Furthermore, just as there are various ways to make an organic product serving with mixed greens, meditation is associated with multiple programs. Since the 1960s, when a popular musical group known as "The Beatles" started doing it, one style known as Transcendental Meditation (TM) has gained the distinction.

TM is not a philosophy, a philosophical system, or a way of existence. Instead, it is a methodology for bringing a greater sense of peace into daily life, with the added benefit of being available. If you're searching for more prominence in your everyday life, relief from anxiety, or a way to slow down your thoughts, meditation will aid. It is fair to assume that all of the above-listed causes directly influence our physical health and, more importantly, our weight.

The mantra method during a meditation session is the fundamental distinction that divides transcendental meditation from other forms of therapies. The mantra is likened to a car used to help the mind settle down and find a safe location.

It is the most common and essential form of meditation. However, it is perhaps the most evolved and, in a general sense, unique approach in terms of the reality that its ease of use is dependent on a thorough understanding of the brain and its behavior, as well as the body, and how the two interact during profound meditation, something that is not fully understood in other methodologies. In this way, all that is needed is a limit of 20 minutes, two days per day, sitting in a comfortable position.

Here are several ways to learn TM:

1. Take a seat in a place that is convenient for you. Crossing your arms or legs is not a good idea.
2. Making sure you're wearing your shades. Take some deep breaths to calm the whole body.
3. Close your eyes and open them again. For the entire 20-minute period, your eyes will be in this state.
4. Choose a mantra to repeat in your head.
5. Refocus your thoughts back on the motto if you find your mind wandering.
6. When the timer beeps, softly move your toes and fingertips to get yourself back to reality.
7. You are attempting to open your eyes.
8. Stay for a prolonged period if you do not feel ready to continue on your day.

Indeed, you might consider how TM will assist with weight loss. According to studies on PTSD survivors, as the psyche grows above, the body expresses itself in a much more profound than even profound rest, and it does so much more quickly. Stress activates a unique instrument that is designed to keep our faith intact. Various exercises are logically started in reaction to this pressure:

1. The front piece of the cerebrum, which is responsible for drive power, would be withdrawn.
2. The output of the happy hormone "dopamine" decreases (while the stress hormone "cortisol" rises).
3. People who are feeling a lot of tension have difficulty turning into their bodies' natural needs.

Growing above is essentially the opposite perception of pressure, and it can have the opposite consequences in this sense. The body's resulting equilibrium allows it to increase profound rest (beyond rest), through which it can disintegrate all its worst anxieties accumulated as a result of life's most heinous injuries. When we become more revived and renewed due to our mediation practice, we can undergo numerous emotional upgrades in various areas of our lives.

Eating With Purpose

We feed without thought. The main reason for our discomfort with food and diet is that we have forgotten how to be available when eating. Careful feeding is the process of being open to how the food we consume affects our bodies, emotions, brains, and everything else about our environment. Our understanding of what to drink, how to eat, how well to eat, and why we eat what we eat increases due to exercise. We are present and relish each chomp as we feed mindfully, integrating all of our faculties to value the nourishment genuinely. We see the presence, noises, scents, and textures of our food, as well as our mind's response to these sensations beyond basic tastes.

The principles of caring relate to healthy eating as well; nevertheless, the concept of careful eating extends beyond the person. It even considers how what you consume affects the whole of the planet. When we feed with this level of comprehension and understanding, we can encounter gratitude and empathy emotions. As a result, conscientious feeding is essential to ensuring nourishment sustainability for who and what is yet to come. We are persuaded to choose foods that are both good for our health and good for the environment.

The reality that the bulk of get-healthy programs struggle in the long term is astounding. After a few years, almost 85 percent of obese people who lose weight return to or exceed their initial weight. Binge dining, passionate eating, outdoor sitting, and eating for nourishment longings have also been attributed to weight gain and weight loss following good weight loss. Continuous exposure to tension will often play a significant role in overeating and gaining weight. The destructive emotions associated with eating may be replaced with mindfulness, increased poise, and optimistic feelings by improving how you think about food. When destructive eating patterns are tackled, the chances of maintaining long-term weight loss increase.

Mindful Eating: A Step-by-Step Guide

1. Keep an eye on our shopping list

Shopping mindfully – ordering healthy foods that are distributed and packaged promptly – is an essential part of the preparation. You'll learn about mindful eating because whole grains are more complex and heavenly than you already knew.

2. Learn how to feed more slowly.

Eating steadily does not have to imply limiting yourself. Overall, it's a good idea to educate yourself and your families that food isn't a competition. Making an effort to enjoy and make the best of your diet is probably the most helpful thing you can do. You'll know that you've finished and you'll bite your food more and, as a result, eat it more quickly, and you'll notice flavors you may have skipped in some way.

3. Eat Just When It's Necessary

Finding the perfect spot between being enthusiastic and greedy to the point where you need to breathe in a dinner may take some practice. Also, pay attention to the body and understand the difference between being mentally hungry and genuinely hungry. If you miss meals, you can be too desperate to get anything into your stomach that your priority becomes filling the vacuum rather than making the most of your food.

4. Respect The Senses

The overwhelming majority of people equate food with flavor, and sometimes people consume so carelessly that their taste buds are put to use. Whatever the case might be, feeding benefits a more extensive range of senses than just taste. Consider shading, surface, smell, and the noises that different foods create when preparing, serving, and consuming them. Take a stab at separating any one of the fixings, especially seasonings, as you bite into your nourishment. To offer your sense of touch a boost, eat with your fingertips. The overall experience becomes considerably more enriching when bringing in different faculties.

5. Keep Distractions to a Minimum

Our everyday lives are filled with interruptions, and it's famous for families to snack when the TV is on, or one relative is fiddling with their iPhone. Consider having family supper time, which should ideally be shared, a hardware-free space. This does not imply that you can eat alone in peace; careful dining may be a wonderful shared experience. It means that you can not feed in front of the screen, when walking, at the monitor, on the cell, or elsewhere. Dining in front of the television is a national pastime; nevertheless, note how easily it promotes reckless eating.

6. When You're Whole, Stop

The thing with incredible nutrition is that it's impossible to resist consuming when it's too good. Eating steadily will make you feel satisfied before overeating, but it's still vital to maintain track of section size and listen to your body for signals that it's had enough. Gorging may sound fantastic at the moment, but it is uncomfortable a short time later and is usually not good for the body. With a bit of practice, you'll be able to find the sweet spot of consuming plenty but not too much.

Careful feeding should not have to be a feat of superhuman concentration, but just a simple pledge to acknowledge, consider, and, most significantly, enjoy the food you consume every day. It can be drilled to help with mixed greens or ice cream, doughnuts, or tofu and eaten at home or college. While the center turns out to be how you consume more than what you eat, you will find that your feelings on what you need to eat improve dramatically as well.

A Means to Lose Weight

This is a kind of reflection skill that you don't just improve over time. It needs preparation, and there will be moments that you fail to eat mindfully, starting from the beginning and finishing with the end.

A Mindful Eating Guide

Individuals who need to be careful regarding food and nutrition should: • Examine their internal information about food — various tastes

- Embrace explicit sustenance inclinations without judgment or self-analysis • Exercise experience with the signs of their bodies starting to feed and refusing to eat.

Principles of Mindful Eating in General

Rebecca J. Frey, Ph.D., and Laura Jean Cataldo, RN, propose a methodology for mindful eating focused on the following core values: Pay attention to the body's intrinsic hunger and satiety signals. Identify personal reasons for mindless feedings, such as peer pressures, unique feelings, and explicit foods.

Here are a few hints to get you started.

- I am starting with only one meal. Any current proclivity necessitates any initial expenditure. Making careful eating practices regularly can be challenging. You should, though, practice for just one dinner or even a portion of a supper. Try to concentrate on the hunger signs and food preferences before you begin feeding, or sink into feelings of satiety at the end of the arrangement — these are fantastic ways to initiate a schedule concerning consideration.

- Place or switching off your phone in a specific location to remove display disturbances. Place aside some mood killers, such as the TV and computer, as well as something else that could distract you from feeding, such as books, magazines, and newspapers. Give the feast until you give it your full attention.
- •When you first begin this activity, pay attention to your viewpoint and your mood. Perceive that there are no correct or wrong approaches to feed, only varying food context knowledge levels. Concentrate concentration on your feeding sensations. If you realize your mind has drifted, softly put it back to the eating awareness.
- This exercise will engage all of the senses. There are several options to consider. Attempt to study a single food item with all of the reasons involved. Consider the scents, surfaces, hues, and flavors when you place food in your mouth. When you cautiously bite each nibble, try to notice how the food varies.
- Take as much time as you like. Eating carefully means taking a step back and encouraging your stomach hormones to warn your brain that you've had plenty before overindulging. It's a great way to prevent the fork from shifting between bites. You'll also be in a better place to enjoy your dining experience, particularly if you're with friends and family.

On the other hand, formal meals would generally take a lower priority in terms of active lives for the general population.

Instead, suppertime is an excuse to attempt to accomplish any of the million tasks one by one.

From the field to the fork — it will help you regulate your appetite, make healthier food decisions, and even appreciate your meals more crisply and perfectly. Take these moves to make the next dinner conscious.

The Most Effective Way to Begin Eating With Intention

First and foremost, feed before you buy. We've always been in the position. You head to the store with a grumbling stomach. When you walk down the halls, those power bars and microwaveable suppers immediately appear tempting. "Shopping will, in general, cut us off from our increasingly talented aspirations of eating in a manner that searches useful for the body while we're overly ravenous," says Dr. Rossy. So, even though you don't have a bottomless appetite to eat, take a healthy snack or a light dinner before leaving home. That way, rather than being driven by hunger or a blood sugar drop, the food decisions can be deliberate as you go shopping.

Stage 2: Make Healthier Food Decisions. If you start worrying about where your food comes from, you'll want healthier food for you, the world, and the people involved in the growing phase. Meredith Klein, an astute cooking instructor, and Pranaful's creator, are portrayed. "While you're in the store, concentrate on the origins of nourishment," Klein demonstrates. "Wishes to determine if it was developed in this country or elsewhere, and seeks to learn about pesticides that might have been applied to or presented to people who were growing food." Make several trips to the own ranchers' market, where the majority of the food is grown locally, if you may, she advises.

Stage 3: Take pleasure in the planning phase. "Value the method more than treating it as an errand or something you have to hurry through before having ready sustenance." Food shopping may be a lot of fun if you purchase products that you believe can help you feel great and nourish your body.

"Just feed," says the fourth level. This is what we do now and then, as plain as it sounds: "just chew." "People sometimes eat while doing various activities, such as looking at their tablets, TVs, computers, and books, as well as mingling," claims Dr. Rossy. "While careful feeding can happen while you're doing other things, aim just to feed' wherever possible." She goes on to say that focusing on the food you're consuming without being preoccupied will help you notice flavors you may not have seen before. Yummy!

Step 4: Put your utensils on the table. When you've finished dining, place your dishes and silverware away right away. This is a warning to yourself that you've got plenty to feed (it tends to be much a bit tough to accept). "You have a charge out of each chomp that way," Klein suggests, "because you're concentrating on the nibble that's in your mouth right now rather than setting up the next one."

Chew, Chew, Chew The Meal at Stage 6. Biting your food is incredibly necessary, and not only because you don't want to be shocked. "When we consume our food with caution, we help the body absorb it more quickly and satisfy a larger portion of our nutritional needs," Dr. Rossy notes. Furthermore, we would not advise you about how much you have consumed the nourishment. On the other side, it indicates chewing before the food is well separated – it would more definitely require longer than a few short bites.

Check-in on Your Hunger at Stage 7. When you consume mindlessly, such as when supper time transforms into prime time to make up for missed time with Netflix or when you get your supper in a hurry, you sometimes ignore the message that your body gives you through the meal. The one that illuminates you as you get to feel whole at the end of the day. Dr. Rossy recommends finishing dinner and checking in on the craving rate. "Keep eating in case there's any uncertainty," she says. "If you're not hungry yet, preserve the food for another day, manure it, or even throw it out." Those remains may be used to create an excellent care dinner the next day.

Last but not least, we understand that sit-down, fully tuned-in mealtimes are not always practical. If you don't have time to complete all seven stages, try to meet one or two every meal. "If you just have a short amount of time," Klein advises, "try to dedicate yourself to food." "Set down your tablet, glance away from the computer, and just be there—no matter how little time you have."

Chapter 7; Daily Weight Loss Meditation

Before you start using meditations to help you burn weight, you must first ensure that you have adequately prepared yourself for your mediation sessions. Each meditation will begin with you entering a deep state of relaxation, followed by directed hypnosis, and ending with you waking from this state of relaxation. If performed right, you can move through the phases of a new attitude and changed actions due to the session.

Make sure you have a private room where you can meditate to better plan for your meditation encounter. You want your meditation time to be as uninterrupted as possible, so you don't wake up. You can be sure that you are relaxed with the room you would be in, in addition to providing a private space. You should lie down or do this meditation before bed with any of the reflections I'll post so that the knowledge settles in as you sleep. Others would need you to sit straight, preferably with your legs crossed on the floor or your feet planted on the floor while seated in a chair. Staying in a sitting posture can help you stay awake and motivated, particularly during morning meditations. Instead of feeling inspired, lying down during these meditations earlier in the day can drain your energy and leave you exhausted. As a consequence, you might find yourself operating against your interests.

These meditations would provide a visualization exercise; however, if visualization is challenging for you in general, you should listen. The aim here is to retain as open a mind as possible to remain sensitive to the knowledge given by these directed meditations.

Besides all of the above, you will improve your meditations by listening to soft music, using a cushion or a small blanket, and dressing in casual, comfortable clothes. You want to find these events as enjoyable as possible such that you look forward to them and participate in them daily. Also, the calmer and at ease you are, the more responsive you would be to the knowledge conveyed to you through each meditation.

An Easy Weight Loss Meditation to Do Every Day

This is a beautiful, easy meditation to do regularly. It's a simple meditation that won't take you more than 15 minutes to finish, and it'll give you plenty of inspiration to stick to your weight-loss plan every day. Every day, set aside time in your morning routine to do this easy ritual weight loss meditation. If you feel your energy waning or your attitude regressing, you can complete it at any time during the day. After a while, you should notice that using it only once a day is sufficient.

Since you'll be performing this meditation first thing in the morning, make sure you're sitting up straight and with a straight spine so you can remain engaged and awake for the period. If you lay down or get too relaxed during your meditation, you can feel more sleepy rather than more alert. This meditation can, in theory, result in increased energy and enhanced fat-burning abilities in your body.

Begin by softly shutting your eyes and concentrating on your breathing. I want you to keep track of the following five breaths as you do so, slowly and deliberately lengthening them to help you calm as fully as possible. Breathe into the count of five and out to the count of seven with each breath. One, two, three, four, five, six, seven, beginning with the next breath in, one, two, three, four, five, six, seven, one, two, three, four, five, six, seven, one, two, three, four, five, six, seven, one, two, three, four, five, six, 1, two, three, four, five, six, seven, one, two, three, four, five, six, seven, one, two, three, four, five, six, seven, one, two, three, four, five, six, seven, one, two, three, four, five 1, two, three, four, five, six, seven, one, two, three, four, five, six, seven, one, two, three, four, five, six, seven, one, two, three, four, five, six, seven, one, two, three, four, five, six, seven, one, two 1, two, three, four, five, six, seven, one, two, three, four, five, six, seven, one, two, three, four, five, six, seven, one, two, three, four, five, six, seven, one, two, three, four, five, six, seven, one, two 1, two, three, four, five, six, seven, one, two, three, four, five, six, seven, one, two, three, four, five, six, seven, one, two, three, four, five, six, seven, one, two, three, four, five, six, seven, one, two, three, four

I want you to get that consciousness into your body now that you're beginning to feel more comfortable. To start, pay attention to your feet. Visualize any tension or worry melting away from your feet when you sense your feet relax profoundly. Now pay attention to your thighs. When your legs begin to relax fully, feel any tension or anxiety melt away. Then, when you become more conscious of your glutes and pelvis, encourage any tension or worry about fading away as they relax entirely literally. Now become aware of your whole torso, causing all stress or worry to melt away while it entirely rests. Then pay attention to the shoulders, sides, wrists, and toes. Enable your shoulders, spine, paws, and fingers to relax fully, releasing tension and concern. Allow the anxiety and respect in your stomach, back, and face to dissipate. When any stress or worry fades away, note how your spine, back, and front relax.

Please take a minute to imagine the room in front of you while you ease further into this state. Imagine yourself standing in front of you, staring down at yourself. See every inch of your body when it stands in front of you right now, casually observing yourself. While you're at it, consider which areas of your body you'd like to lose weight in so you can build a better, more muscular body for yourself. Visualize the importance of these parts of the body melting away as you build out a healthy, leaner, and stricter body underneath it. When you try to imagine yourself being a happier and more energetic version of yourself, note how easily the excess fat falls away.

Now think what you might be like if you were a better, leaner version of yourself. Imagine yourself going through your everyday life as though you were a healthier version of yourself. What would you eat if you were in this situation? Where and how will you work out? What will you do in your free time? What are your thoughts on yourself? When you associate with the people around you, such as your relatives and coworkers, how different do you feel? How does it sound to be a better, cleaner version of yourself?

Consider how different your life is now that your fat has melted away for a few minutes. Observe how natural it is for you to eat these nutritious meals, as well as how easy it is for you to manage your cravings and indulgences while you do. Note how convenient it is for you to work out and how it sounds more like a relaxing activity than a job. I feel like you love life more now that the fatty fats that were dragging you down and causing health problems have vanished. Remember how straightforward it was to get here and how simple it would be to preserve your wellbeing and fitness while you create more and better decisions for yourself and your body.

When you make these better decisions, you'll realize how much you love your body and how much you feel for yourself. Take note about how and meal and workout seems like an act of self-care rather than a chore you're compelled to do. Consider how good it feels to do something about yourself. And the benefit of your health.

When you're ready, take a picture of yourself and submit it out as far as you can until it's nothing but a spec in your field of consciousness. So, release it into the ether, hoping that your subconscious mind can hang on to this image of yourself and focus on getting it into the present life regularly.

Now, return to your current position in your body. Feel more energized, inspired, and optimistic about participating in events that can boost your wellbeing and help you burn fat. Keep on to the visualization and those thoughts about yourself as you plan to go through your day, and believe that you will have this great moment in your life. You've got this!

Fat Burning Meditation

This fat-burning meditation is a basic 30-minute meditation that allows you to see the fat cells shrinking into smaller and smaller cells until they disappear entirely. Reflections are supposed to further guide the subconscious mind about how to deal with your body so that you can continue to get a happier and healthier body by focusing on certain forms of hypnosis. When you deliberately drag your subconscious awareness into specific practices, it allows it to continue doing so on its own, particularly when you are not in hypnosis.

This is an ideal meditation to do one to three days a week during the day or bedtime. They claim that meditating right before bedtime may be especially helpful because you're contemplating. Simultaneously, your subconscious mind is busier, and your conscious mind is only about to fall asleep. During this time, you are more likely to feel the degree of calm and receptivity that your subconscious mind needs to digest the adjustments you wish to create entirely.

Enable yourself to close your eyes and drift into a deep state of relaxation to begin this meditation. Each - breath, note how you're calming deeper and deeper and how you're slipping into a beautiful form of calmness. To help you deepen your relaxation, I will lead you through a practice that will enable you to achieve the most profound degree of ease possible. I want you to see yourself standing at the top of a flight of stairs to do this. I want you to picture yourself going down the flight of stairs, one step at a time, as I count down from one to ten. Visualize yourself calming more and deeper with each action you take until you're in a deep state of relaxation and ready to begin a hypnotic visualization session.

When you count down from ten, imagine yourself taking a walk down the stairs. Take notice of the environment, including the color of the walls, the form of the bottom level, and any decorations that might be present. Step down again with nine, and you'll find that you're moving closer to the bottom of the flight of stairs. When you walk down to the eighth step, notice how your relief doubles with each step. As you descend lower and lower down the stairs, note how your view will be shifting around you going down to the seventh stair. Now descend to the sixth stairwell. Drop down to the fifth stair when you're finished, feeling the relaxation double when you fall deeper and deeper into a state of relaxation and calmness. Now descend to the fourth stairwell. When you walk down to the third stair, you can see a chair come into focus when you look ahead. As you descend the second stair, you note that the chair seems to be very comfortable, and you can't wait to sit in it and feel the relaxation increase threefold as you descend the first stair and then exit the staircase.

Imagine yourself going up to the chair and sitting in it until you reach the bottom of the stairs. You'll notice that this chair is the most comfortable chair you've ever sat in and that when you fall into it, the whole state relaxes ten times deeper. Feel yourself calming down to the point that you can simply fade away in this room.

Observe your awareness shifting inward towards your body while you remain there. Draw your attention down into your fat cells as your awareness shifts inward. Consider how each cell is hugging your body, holding you safe and relaxed in your current state. Take notice of how each cell is secure in its work and sits proudly in its location. When you study one of these fat cells, note that they are not there to damage or kill you, but simply that they feel they are allowed to be there. They think they are performing a vital role in your life.

I'd like you to take one up in your hand while you get your awareness closer to these cells. Remember the tiny round cell in your palm, which is proudly fulfilling a role in your life. Thank the cell for what it has provided for you while you keep it, and let it realize that you no longer need its assistance. Feel the cell diminishing down until it vanishes between your palms when you cup it between your lips.

Take up a new cell and keep it in your palms once more. Thank it from the bottom of your heart for fulfilling its mission and inform it that you no longer need its assistance. As you cup it in your hands and shrink it down until it vanishes, wish it well.

Continue doing this for your fat cells, picking them up, thanking them for their help, and then shrinking them back in your hands until they disappear entirely. Allow each fat cell to realize that it is no longer required and that you appreciate what it has given you up to this point in your life. Allow your remaining cells to understand that you now need less fat in your body to reclaim your wellbeing and begin to feel better.

When you hit the edge of the fat cells, you'll find that no fat cells are remaining. You see healthy cells that help the body perform vital functions like cell regrowth, digestion, and circulation. Enable yourself to shed this outlook when you return your mind to your body. Express deep appreciation for every single cell in your body and the job it is doing. When you return to space where you rest, see your consciousness extending past the scale of your tiny cells and returning to the awareness of yourself. As you raise your eyes and feel new in your body, feel yourself waking from your meditation.

See how, even if some of your fat cells exist, you can almost see them vanishing when you go through your everyday life from now on. Please continue to show appreciation for each cell and what it has achieved to help you live and encourage it to fade away comfortably when you return to a state of poor health.

Chapter 8; Power of Affirmation

Offer yourself the gift of thinking power every day. The idea that your perceptions build your social situations and conditions is at the core of thought power. Any part of your current existence, including your relationships, wealth, fitness, and self-image, is the product of your most prevalent thoughts and the feelings, emotions, and values they create.

You are not your circumstances; you are the maker of your events, whether desirable or unwanted. Accepting the fact that your thoughts build your situation by their infinite imaginative force, the best approach to creative thinking consciousness is to get the truth that through becoming mindful of the most normal thoughts in your head, you will decide which thoughts/seeds to nurture and care about, thus altering your reality or circumstance.

Look inside yourself to build thinking consciousness, and the reality starts in your head. You can only construct knowledge of thought by becoming conscious of your thoughts. You can alter the energy in particular places of your existence by becoming mindful of the power generated by specific, simple ideas.

Thoughts are the root of your prevailing attitudes, values, and mental mindset (the situation), which is why you must become mindful of them lest you attract unsightly conditions, behaviors, and beliefs, and therefore a hideous existence that never enables you to fulfill your maximum capacity, which you realize you have enough of.

Per day, the typical person has between 6,000 and 70,000 feelings. Thoughts are not equal, and some of them are transient, something we may only refer to as "mind musings." The most important senses that can transform your life are how you bind the most emotional power and worry about most often.

Thinking mindfulness is a learned habit that requires you to practice how to strike a balance between obsessively tracking all of your feelings — including brief ones that have little bearing on your existence — and awareness of your most habitual thoughts.

Thinking consciousness does not mean obsessing about every thought; rather, it implies becoming conscious of your habitual feelings, since, as previously said, only the ideas you replicate and to which you bind emotions to have the power to alter your existence. You may use curated thoughts (affirmations) to change every viewpoint and part of your existence or situation as you begin to understand and adopt these thoughts accordingly (including how you view them).

A significant portion of our thoughts is automatic. Because of the many ideas the human mind encounters each day, science predicts that 95-99 percent of our thoughts and actions are involuntary.

Since the mind is a professional automation system that automates to conserve brainpower, it is possible to construct a drastically different truth than the one you want if you are not mindful of your thinking. For example, whether you desire a better career or a new home but your more popular thoughts or feelings regarding such ventures are pessimistic, or you think you are undeserving of certain things, your situations can only improve once you change your thoughts and, as a consequence, your beliefs and behaviors.

The Tool for Improving Thinking Consciousness

Perception is the first step in developing mind comprehension. Our most common impressions are conditioned feelings that contribute to behaviors; how we "react" regarding a situation is determined by our thoughts and perceptions.

It's important and set aside time to listen to your feelings if you choose to become more aware of them. There are several ways to do this, but a reflection, encouragement, and artistic imagery are the most successful.

Meditation is a technique for calming the

Spending 5 minutes in your mind and being mindful of the feelings, desires, behaviors, and values that flow through it at every given moment is a gift.

Aim to relax for the next 5 minutes (how much time you invest depends on your preferences). Relaxing your thinking mind eliminates the pathways between your conscious and subconscious brains, making it possible to embed affirmations into your subconscious and unconscious minds.

Practicing breath and mindfulness therapy is the simplest way to calm and covertly become more conscious of the most ordinary emotions.

Breathe in for a count of four, paying attention to the nuance of your breath as you inhale. Take notice of the vibrations you experience when you keep your breath for a count of four.

Take notice of the feelings when you exhale to a count of four: How air travels up the bronchial tube and erupts in a hot puff from your mouth or nose. Imagine the hot breath carrying your stress, fear, and pain with it when you exhale; picture this as vividly as possible, as it will make you calm profoundly. Keep your breath for four counts before restarting the sequence and repeating before you are comfortable.

This breathing method, also known as 4-part breathing, stimulates the parasympathetic nervous system responsible for rest, relaxing, and digestion. When enabled, this mechanism causes the thinking mind to relax.

You will then begin the process of being mindful of your stream of consciousness and noticing the most normal thoughts about various facets of your life while you start to relax.

Mindfulness, which is described as the willingness to sit with one's thoughts without analyzing them, may help you become more mindful of your most popular thoughts. Being aware of these emotions, mainly when they apply to essential aspects of your life, will help you identify which values, attitudes, and mindsets you need to alter to make meaningful changes.

Note: Affirmations are a transformative method in a toolbox that includes several other resources required to accomplish a project effectively (perhaps a goal, desire, or change of belief).

The bulk of unsuccessful affirmation tests fail due to a misalignment between the affirmation replicated and one's views or emotions towards the affirmation topic.

For example, utilizing an assertion like "I am wealthy" while you are broke is unlikely to succeed because you first take steps to help you create wealth and then court thoughts that lead you to think you are deserving of that wealth.

Bear in mind that the world reacts to the sounds in your words when you practice regular affirmations (the ones you use to word your affirmations). The terms are not recognized by it. Simply placed, the vibrational force you draw into your life/circumstances is determined by how you feel regarding the reinforcement (and its associated region of your life).

Affirmations are designed to help you experience the vibrational energy/feeling you like to know such that the world picks up on it and draws related vibrational energies to it.

Journaling, Affirmations, and Critical Thought

Another powerful method to build thinking consciousness is to use affirmations, particularly those made for the fundamental goal of transforming your life. Claims are intended to help you adjust the vibrational rhythm, feelings, and perceptions regarding particular facets of your existence. It is difficult to calculate the present vibrational force, let alone alter it, without thinking knowledge.

It's a good idea to take more time in your feelings while contributing to a specific region of your life before you start writing affirmations. Thinking of the tension that arises as you worry about your life's particular aspects is a critical way to do this. This can expose the most typical thinking habits in that region of your life; you may also take things a step further and journal your feelings in a stress log, one of the most potent thought awareness resources.

Stress journaling (and journaling in general) helps you keep track of your stressful feelings over time, giving you a snapshot of the most frequent stress-inducing. These negative thoughts pump out negative vibrational energy into the world. Through this knowledge, you will develop customized affirmations that you trust and have the power to transform the feelings you associate with those aspects of your existence.

Often bear in mind that, while affirmations are a potent weapon, they cannot be used alone. It helps to know as much as you can about your life aspect you wish to improve while writing affirmations. This knowledge enables you to discover the values, patterns, and related vibrational energies associated with that region of your existence, making it easy to utilize affirmations to effect massive improvement.

Thinking knowledge helps you to doubt your more normal feelings regarding a particular feature of your existence and, as a result, consider more rationally.

Fear is also the root of pessimistic feelings. You get to see the root source of the negativity of your life as you journal them. The method of questioning and confronting your negative feelings gets more apparent as you become conscious of what you are thinking and experiencing.

For example, you may question the validity of any of the negative/stressing thoughts you journaled and thereby decide whether the thinking has any value by doing so. Coincidentally, by questioning negative thoughts, beliefs, and assumptions in this manner, it will be easier to challenge feelings of inadequacy, worries, and anxieties over your abilities and other people's reactions to you and your work.

Journaling (both tension journaling and general journaling) is one of the most potent ways to raise thinking comprehension. Every day, want to practice doing that (preferably twice a day: Once in the morning and once in the evening as you wind down for the night).

Affirmation for Weight Loss

Each person's soul has its form of meditation. Likely, the way I meditate isn't for you. Your approach would not work for me, either. Some people aren't making the best out of their practice, and they aren't meditating correctly for them. If you don't have access to a yoga master, you'll have to go deep inside yourself and attempt to pull your meditation from the darkest recesses of your core. For a novice, this may be tough. Look deep inside yourself and see whether you can hear a sound, have a feeling or have a concept. If that's the case, pursue that speech, that thought, and see if it brings you joy or peace. It must be a sensation in which there are no queries, difficulties, or suspicions. And when you get the feeling, would you be able to say whether the sound you heard is the authentic inner voice that will support you on your spiritual path.

Meditation Preparation

Until you begin meditating, you should be aware of specific essential considerations. First and foremost, make sure you've taken care of all physical criteria (hunger, thirst, etc.). Be sure you're not ill because you'll have a hard time getting into the correct frame of mind and staying relaxed if you are. In ideal conditions, the location where you want to meditate should be relaxing and unobtrusive. To avoid being distracted, switch off all electrical gadgets that can cause you to become distracted. To meditate, lie down in a relaxed position. You may do this by sitting in a chair or the lotus pose or posture or lying down on a bed, but the latter is more likely to result in sleep. Other people like to meditate outside rather than at home. Other creatures or disturbances do not bother us. We can meditate while listening to soothing music but switch it off if it distracts or disturbs us. It's good if you need quiet or the sound of nature. If you like to listen to music, make sure you choose the correct kind; certain music will help you into alpha, and others will help you beta. You must be able to relax when listening to music.

Let's have a look at how we can meditate and the various available approaches!

You may start by using the color visualization tool. For 5 seconds, picture the shades red-orange-yellow-green-blue-violet-purple. The order of the colors progresses from higher to lower frequency. If a color is brighter, you might display artifacts with that color. If you excel, try a more advanced simulation technique. Consider not only stain and form but also landscape, which provides one with a sense of well-being. The first thing we remember when learning meditation is how to breathe correctly: Inhaling for a couple of seconds, then fully exhaling, waiting a few minutes, and then breathing again. We go through this time and again. Take a brief break before exhaling and the following inhalation if necessary. Never do something that might endanger your health or your lungs. When completing breathing exercises, the first thing to consider is purity. You will efficiently purify the air if you can feel while breathing that the breath comes directly from Heaven, Innocence.

To meditate more efficiently, you must strengthen your concentration. What's much more is that it can happen on its own when you're contemplating. Everything you have to do now meditates, meditate, and meditate some more. You can pick which part of your body to concentrate on; make sure it's the one that feels yours. If you're a total novice, concentrate on a small point on your body, such as your eye, nose, or fingertip, rather than your hands, arms, or legs. The concentration will be higher if the point is lower (Ware, 2014).

The countdown method is one of the most common. Slowly count down 5-10-20 one by one to begin to move into a more profound condition. Here's how to do it:

- 10 - I feel relaxed,
- 9 - My body gradually relaxes,
- 8 - I am in a deeper state of consciousness,
- 7 - All stress leaves me,
- 6 - I don't have any tension,
- 5 - I feel like my whole body is relaxed,
- 4 - I am gradually entering a calmer state of consciousness,
- 3 - My mind is still, and I let go of all thoughts,
- 2 - I achieve inner happiness,

If you attempt hypnosis, you'll most definitely experience the so-called fixed viewing technique, which allows you to stare at a particular spot. We reach a deeper state of consciousness during hypnosis because we are meditating in a way (Mindful word, n. d.).

You'll find yourself combining the strategies listed above as you develop.

The brain is in a different state of mind than average during meditation. Several degrees can be differentiated depending on how far we travel. The Greek letters Alpha, Beta, Theta, and Delta, are used to describe each consciousness step. Per state of consciousness is correlated with a specific brain frequency. And during meditation, the subject may be studied with the appropriate diagnostic equipment. What are our current understandings of Beta? On an average of 14-20 Hz, this is the natural state of consciousness we spend our waking days. In this state, we are conscious of the usual physical environment, like function, research, etc. When we are under a lot of tension, our brains will emit much higher frequencies. What does it mean to be in the Alpha state? It operates at a frequency of 7-14 Hz and is also known as a superconscious condition. So, we're still awake, but we're in a comfortable situation, and a sense of peace surrounds us. People are more open to feedback while they are in this condition. We are typically in this condition while we meditate. Our brains operate at 4-7 Hz while we are in the Theta process. The so-called shamanic journeys take place in this condition of superficial sleep. We are in Delta, which has a frequency of 1-4 Hz, while we sleep profoundly.

Following the planning, we attempt to reach a changed state of consciousness using one or more of the aforementioned approaches. Try to rid the head of all such distracting emotions when doing so. The most challenging task for most people is to eliminate the intrusive feelings that continually divert their attention. What would we do to prevent this from happening?

It's like telling a monkey or a pigeon not to bother you if you try to manipulate your mind with your human will. You can see that that isn't feasible. To quiet the intellect, we must enlist the aid of a higher force. This force is the soul's life. You must get the soul's light into your core. Imagine them as two rooms: one for the heart and one for the mind. The intellect space is now dim, filthy, and refuses to open to the sun.

On the other hand, the spirit lives in the heart space, which is still exposed to light. If you reflect and meditate on the truth within your core rather than your intellect, the fact can come to the fore. You should reach your mind room to enlighten it if you have already rooted yourself in your core and the illumination of the soul has saturated you.

It's helpful to remember that every optimistic comment may be seen as evidence because everyone can quickly make their targeted affirmations. You may use generic claims, but you would be best off coming up with individual statements tailored to your situation. These affirmations' efficacy may be significantly improved by utilizing them at the correct time, right after our negative comment, and by remembering to provide immediate input on our excellent work, such as, "You achieved, as you can see! This will be the case in the future!" We will deliberately manipulate our subconscious by utilizing affirmations. We will guide our whole life in a better direction by modifying our actions, behaviors, and attitudes (Hussain & Bhutan, 2010).

Boost Your Self-Belief

The shift will come quickly when constructive reinforcements are used. However, don't get disappointed if it takes longer than you planned because you'll continue to work every day to see progress. The amount of time depends on how firmly we believe, what we want, and how significant our priorities are. It is important to stress that it can only succeed if we entirely remove our heads' harmful feelings. I advocate using constructive motivation in the mornings, so we prefer to start the day with a positive outlook, and we tend to be more stressed about our issues in the afternoons.

Why Can Constructive Reinforcement Be Used?

Select quick thoughts that reinforce each other. When we go over these again, keep quiet. Concentrate on the origins of terms that occur frequently. If you believe what you're doing, you must believe that your wishes have been satisfied or are in the process of being fulfilled.

Among the statements, stop utilizing offensive terms. Instead of saying, "I'm not overweight," say, "I'm at my perfect weight." As a result, instead of pessimistic thoughts, the imagination creates a constructive one. It's important to remember that confirmation statements are written in the present tense, not the future. We use the current version of "I am glad" instead of "I would be happy." At a time, just use one form of reinforcement. Concentrating on a single task can yield more efficient and quicker performance. You must be able to see and sense your needs to engage them in your life. Whatever the current condition is, emotional tuning is essential.

Affirmation for Feeling Better

In the second half of this segment, we'll look at more than 300 affirmations that will help you lose weight, enhance your fitness, and feel happier in general. You can use these affirmations just as they are, or you can tweak them to suit your own beliefs. If you should decide to revise them, make sure they directly represent what you need to say to shift the views to more supportive and less restrictive views.

Self-Control Affirmations

Self-control is a crucial skill to possess, and lacking it will contribute to habits that make weight reduction more difficult. If you're having trouble with self-control, the affirmations below will help you adjust any self-control values you have so you can treat diet, fitness, weight reduction, and nutrition in general with healthy beliefs.

- I am self-disciplined.
- My superpower is my willpower.
- I am in control of my actions.
- I have the authority to make a decision.
- I am committed to fulfilling my aims.
- I am good because I am self-disciplined.
- I am worthy of persevering in the face of adversity.
- I am open to solving barriers.
- My mind is efficient, disciplined, and solid.
- My interests are within my influence.
- I have a success mentality.
- Every day, I strengthen my discipline.
- I am naturally self-discipline.
- I have a lot of self-control.
- I am effective because I am in command.
- Every day, it becomes simpler for me to excel.
- I see myself as a self-disciplined, successful person.
- I have a natural capacity to retain self-control.
- It's as normal as breathing to exercise self-control.
- I am in command of my emotions.
- I am in control of my actions.
- I'm confident in my ability to persevere.
- I can summon self-control anytime I need it.

- My appetite is more significant than my self-control.
- I have a tremendous amount of self-control.
- In either case, I can comfortably retain my self-control.
- I'm a stickler for seeing it out until the finish.
- I believe I should depend on myself to make healthy decisions.
- Making good decisions is easy for me.
- I have no trouble controlling my urges.
- My natural condition is that of self-control.
- I'll keep going before I accomplish my purpose.
- I'm beginning to enjoy the sensation of self-control.
- I believe myself to be a good person.
- My willpower is unbreakable.
- I have a substantial degree of self-control.
- I am a self-disciplined person.
- I achieve every target I set for myself.
- I am a rather deliberate human.
- My self-control strengthens with each passing day.
- I'm cultivating a good sense of self-discipline.
- My self-discipline is the key to my performance.
- I am a powerful and competent person.
- I'm committed to fulfilling my fitness objectives.
- One of my most significant assets is self-control.
- I am absolutely in charge of the scenario.
- I believe I am capable of completing this mission.
- I am capable and self-aware.
- Through self-control and appreciation, I will go on.

- o I still carry through with what I think I'm going to do.
- o I have the determination to succeed.
- o I will trust myself to make the best decision.
- o I have confidence in my willingness to persevere.
- o I'm becoming better by the day.
- o I make my decisions with self-control.
- o I'm dedicated to seeing this through.
- o I make careful judgments.
- o I am dedicated to achieving my goals.

Self-Esteem Affirmations

Self-esteem is crucial when it comes to body appearance. Low self-esteem may be both the source and the product of an unfavorable body picture. If you're dissatisfied with how you look and act, it may be that you lack the self-confidence to make a difference, or it could be because of your current health condition. In any case, improving your self-esteem now will help you stay dedicated to your fitness objectives and increase your ability to cultivate a body shape and quality of wellbeing that you find more appealing.

1) I am entitled to a comfortable, stable body and life.
2) I am a one-of-a-kind person.
3) Life is both satisfying and fulfilling.
4) I deserve a body that enables me to see all life has to bring.
5) Right now, I want to be content and safe. My life is excellent.
6) I choose to adopt a balanced lifestyle.
7) I am prosperous now and in the future.
8) Every day, I strive to be the most robust version of myself.

9)   I have the freedom to enjoy my body.
10) I am deserving of a rewarding life experience.
11) I am committed to myself, my marriage, and my general well-being.
12) I am a caring and loving person.
13) I am an enthusiastic and energetic individual.
14) I am entitled to the most excellent possible treatment for my body and well-being.
15) I am a versatile and adaptable person.
16) I enjoy thinking optimistic things about myself and my outward image.
17) I'm surrounded by people who accept me for who I am.
18) My views represent who I am.
19) I surround myself with people who inspire me to be my true self.
20) Every day, I make an effort to be my best self.
21) I can make positive changes in my life.
22) I am worthy of devotion.
23) I have earned the right to feel confident for myself.
24) I have high regard for myself, my body, and my welfare.
25) I have an exclusive proposition for you.
26) I have confidence in myself.
27) I am capable of feeling confident for myself as a whole.
28) I'm involved in improving my self-esteem.
29) I should feel positive about myself when working every day to improve myself.
30) I do display compassion and reverence to myself and my body.
31) I decided to respect myself.
32) I see myself in a positive light.

33) I am in love with myself.
34) I am open to evolving into the most potent iteration of myself.
35) I am pleased with myself and my wishes.
36) I'm concerned about my health, my body, and my overall well-being.
37) It gives me the joy to be committed to myself.
38) I openly applaud myself.
39) People admire me for who I am.
40) I am confident of who I am.
41) I am deserving of a beautiful existence.
42) I am deserving of apparel that flatters my body.
43) Every day, I gain more self-assurance.
44) Thank you so much.
45) I am grateful for my body.
46) My body is committed to me.
47) My body is deserving of good health.
48) I take care of myself by dreaming, sleeping, and doing things that are beneficial for me.
49) My well-being is essential to me.
50) I can enhance my hygiene.
51) I give my body the respect it deserves.
52) I find it a priority to respect and care about myself at all times.
53) When I look at my body, I see it from the eyes of passion.
54) Through the light of passion, I see myself.
55) I'm cool with being in love with myself.
56) My body needs to be at its peak.

Affirmations for a Beautiful Existence

It can be difficult to note that you are terrific at all points of your journey, even the parts you don't like, as we are adjusting the way our bodies appear. Using affirmations that help you affirm your attractiveness will boost your self-esteem, self-confidence, and self-worth and make you feel positive about yourself overall. Furthermore, the more beautiful you sound, the more apt you are to engage in your physical health and beauty, ensuring you would be much more inspired to eat better and workout regularly to lose weight permanently.

1) I am sexy both on the inside and out.
2) The happier I am, the more desirable I am.
3) I am beautiful because I am happy with myself.
4) My skin is radiant, clear, and stable.
5) My body is stunning.
6) My skin is transparent, smooth, and gentle.
7) I like staring in the mirror and admiring myself.
8) I am a lovely girl.
9) I am thankful for my lovely body.
10) My body is getting more exquisite every day.
11) I am surrounded by natural beauty.
12) My body is enticing.
13) My body is fit and desirable.
14) Being attractive is second nature to me.
15) My body has a natural charm.
16) My body type is attractive.
17) My one-of-a-kind beauty is breathtaking.
18) I have a brilliant sense of design.
19) I handle myself with grace and faith.
20) I am in excellent health.
21) I am a young woman.
22) I'm at home with my skin.
23) It makes me happy to be admired by myself and others.
24) I am stunning just the way I am.
25) My mind, body, and spirit are all stunning manifestations of who I am.
26) I'm happy with myself the way I am.
27) I exude genuine grace.
28) Because life is amazing, I want to laugh and love it.

29) My features are attractive.
30) My faults, though, are beautiful.
31) My aura shines brightly.
32) I'm happy to be as attractive as I am.
33) Everybody will see my charm.
34) Every day, I am becoming more stunning.
35) I'm in an excellent mood.
36) Every day, my features improve in attractiveness.
37) My appearance increases as I take care of myself.
38) I love myself, and beauty is a product of my inner self-love.
39) I have a natural charm.
40) My body is perfectly perfect.
41) I am stunning in every way.
42) People comment on how attractive I am.
43) I was blessed with natural elegance.
44) I am a one-of-a-kind beauty.
45) I don't judge myself against anyone. I am gorgeous and one-of-a-kind.
46) I am mindful of my natural appearance.
47) I'm confident in my skin.
48) I think what I see in the reflection is lovely.
49) I adore myself completely.
50) I see myself as a wonderful, lovable woman.
51) I am stunning.
52) I accept praises gracefully.
53) I am entitled to be pretty.
54) My inner elegance shines through.
55) I am stunning in every aspect.
56) I am a stunning, radiant woman.
57) I gratefully accept my appearance.
58) I want to be attractive.

Chapter 9; Diet

Dietary adjustment is one of the most daunting facets of weight reduction. Our eating preferences are deeply rooted in our personalities. We get emotions from comfort foods from our youth or foods that are familiar to our taste buds. Furthermore, our eating patterns and interactions are similar to our social habits. Consequently, improving what you consume can sound overwhelming and time-consuming, but it does not have to be. You should make lifestyle adjustments that can help you shed weight while still helping you feel healthier. The key is to stop any dramatic dietary adjustments. Instead of removing those food classes or adding foods to a "do not consume" registry, make subtle adjustments to develop healthier behaviors. You should also be able to eat anything. You won't consume them too much, and if you can find better options, you won't regret them almost as often. It takes some time to adapt to the adjustments, but they will feel natural after a month.

More emphasis should be put on consistency rather than quantities. To consume a balanced diet, you don't have to restrict yourself to four cups of lettuce with a bit of oil. Permit yourself to indulge in the chocolate cake or burger. Choose a smaller piece. Try half or three-quarters of a burger instead of the entire thing. Get the most OK burger you can buy, but quit when you're done rather than pushing yourself to finish. Allow things to taste nice and take pleasure in what you're consuming. To be happy, you don't need a ton of it. You won't continue to consume vast amounts of something if you allow yourself to eat it daily without restriction. You'll be satisfied with only a tiny amount, and it's a simple adjustment to make so you won't feel like you're losing out. Placed, you're setting the standard of the experience ahead of the amount.

Calories can be measured loosely. Know that strict calorie counting will cause you to lose track of your hunger signals.

Thirst signals are essential for weight loss since they can help you differentiate between your appetite, or need to eat, and your hunger, or need to eat. Many individuals neglect their appetite signs due to fad diets or excessive feeding, finding it impossible to differentiate between their physical requirements and mental food urges. Calories alone do not offer a complete image. Your body needs more calories on specific days than on others. For example, if you're cleaning up the kitchen, your body may know that you need more calories, even if your calorie tracking software tells you that you should be consuming the same amount every day. Rather than having to push yourself to finish a specific number every day, listen to your hunger signals and use calories as a supplementary statistic to help you get back in contact with your hunger cues. Be mindful of what you're consuming and why you're eating it, but leave yourself some leeway and hold a loose calorie count.

Don't be stingy about yourself. According to research, depriving yourself of the things you like the most will sabotage your weight reduction efforts. When you divide foods into "poor" and "healthy" ranges, you begin to think in black and white terms. There is no curve when this way of thought is used. Suppose you are entirely correct or completely incorrect. As a result, consuming a slice of cake might lead to eating a bag of chips or drinking a sugary beverage when you think to yourself, "I've already done one poor thing, I may as well do some more until I have to start eating lettuce and celery again tomorrow." This attitude is all too popular, particularly among emotional eaters who use food to cope with many emotions, including depression, boredom, or desire. Deprivation sends the incorrect message to the body, which may cause you to spin.

The secret to and ultimate purpose of mindful eating is to be aware of what you're eating. Mindful eating is a form of meditation that uses your internal energies to help you control your appetite and offer your body everything it wants without worrying too much about it. Mindful eating allows you to feed whatever you like to get everything you want. This practice helps you recognize that no one will eat poorly or appropriately and that everyone's dining experience would be unique. It also encourages you to be present at the moment and deal with the appetite when it arises. When eating mindfully, make decisions that will nourish your body and make you feel healthy. As a result, though diet is essential, indulgence is permitted. Mindful eating is only food. It's just about going back to the fundamentals and breaking the unhealthy association with food. It's just about achieving harmony and equilibrium between your feelings and your appetite. To be conscious, what you have to do is become more knowledgeable of your dietary patterns and when and when you turn to food. Consider whether you're mentally or physically hungry. Finally, select foods that are delicious but still providing the body with the nutrition it needs. You will achieve equilibrium due to this, and you will never have to count calories again!

Fiber is beneficial to your health. Fiber-rich foods are a healthy option for snacking because they sustain you fuller for longer and better control the digestive system. Fiber often decreases the chance of losing weight or gaining more fat, making it an essential weight-loss weapon. Wool is also safe for the heart and reduces your chances of having type 2 diabetes. Consequently, no matter what size you are, it can help you gain weight and be healthy overall. If you plan to increase fiber consumption, do it steadily. Abdominal pain and gassiness may result from eating so much extra fiber at once. Consequently, while the yarn is good for you, your body may require time to adapt to higher amounts. Start adding more fiber-rich items to your diets, such as fruits, berries, beans, and nuts.

You can feel fuller and better by consuming whole grains. They frequently produce a high volume of fiber and, for different purposes, make you feel complete. Foods that have been minimally refined are known as whole foods. Whole food is an almond, while apple sauce is canned food. Since processing will eliminate any of the nutrients and beneficial side effects from the food, the whole apple would provide further health benefits. It isn't to suggest you can't eat refined foods, but attempting to have more whole foods in your diet would mean you receive the nutrition your body needs to perform at its best. Both fruits and vegetables are excellent options. Start consuming the cranberry itself rather than the sugary juice type if you want cranberry juice. Furthermore, whole-grain rice (or whole-grain bread) is preferable to white rice (or whole-grain bread) because it has more nutrients and can satiate you longer than the non-whole grain variety.

Substitute natural sugars for refined sugars. Try a bowl of berries instead of heading for the bowl of ice cream. Few diets demonize fruits because they are rich in sugar, but the advantage of fruits is that they can fill you up and offer nutrition in a way that ice cream can not. The fruit is an outstanding dessert option since it can please your sweet tooth while still holding you hydrated and supplying fiber. Fruits are, above all, valuable natural foods. Fruit, such as apples, has been shown in experiments to help dieters, but don't remove it from your diet. About one out of every ten adults in the United States met the CDC's fruit guidelines. Furthermore, in 2017, three-point-nine million deaths were linked to not eating enough fruits and vegetables worldwide, demonstrating the importance of these foods to your health.

Your mother was right when she advised you to consume your vegetables. They're whole foods that are high in fiber and are nutrient-dense superfoods. Using various vegetables in your diet would mean that you get a broad spectrum of nutrients, growing your appetite, and providing the body with all the nutrients it needs to get through the day. Broccoli, onions, and spinach are also called superfoods since they have too many beneficial nutrients. Vegetables are low in calories and strong in liquids, which lets you remain hydrated in the same way as fruits do.

Keep yourself hydrated. Water's strength is undeniable. People can live for long periods without food than they can without water. As a consequence, you do not underestimate the value of hydration. Often people misinterpret thirst with food, so if you're starving, worry about whether you're dehydrated. According to research, people who drink one glass of water before meals ingest seventy-five calories fewer on average because water serves as an appetite suppressant. With this number in mind, this approach could help you lose eight pounds in a year! Furthermore, simply substituting water for one beverage a day will significantly decrease your calorie intake. Moreover, water helps wash the body, meaning that the body performs correctly and your metabolism stays high, rendering weight loss simpler.

Learn new recipes and expand your culinary horizons. Take advantage of this opportunity to broaden your culinary knowledge and desires. Discover different ways to appreciate and interact with cooking. You should start learning to love cooking right now and avoid depending on take-out or restaurant meals. Find new recipes you like or modify old ones to meet the new requirements. Don't be scared to prepare rich foods. You should consume rich foods while staying balanced! The Mediterranean diet is full of delectable foods and is commonly recognized as one of the healthiest diets possible. The Mediterranean diet, an eating style standard in Southern Europe, decreases the likelihood of cancers and other health conditions such as stroke, high blood pressure, Parkinson's disease, cardiac disease, Alzheimer's disease, and type 2 diabetes.

Optimal Nutrition

People automatically dream about eating well as they think about having a better body. However, consuming nutritious meals does not ensure that you can reach the perfect physique. Although being in the best shape of your life does not always imply that you are eating healthily. To eat healthily, you usually supply the body with enough nutrients to survive properly. To function at its highest, the body needs a certain amount of macronutrients (carbohydrates, proteins, and carbohydrates) and micronutrients (vitamins and minerals). You must fulfill your body's dietary needs to promote optimal health. Losing weight or adding muscle usually is necessary to attain a great body. To lose weight, you must sustain a calorie imbalance, which means your body loses more calories than you consume and drink. Gaining weight necessitates the calorie surplus, in which you eat more calories than the body burns down.

While consuming nutritious foods has several advantages, it is equally necessary to fulfill your exercise target's requirement. For instance, if your goal is to lose weight and consume 10,000 calories of vegetables a day, you eat healthily, drinking a ton of calories to accomplish your goal. As a result, it's better to eat the target weight when maintaining good fitness.

What is the concept of a calorie?

Calories are often mentioned, but what exactly do they imply? A calorie is a unit of energy measurement. The sum of energy in the food you consume is calculated rather than its quantity or weight. When you hear something has 100 calories in that, it's explaining how much energy the body can receive by consuming or consuming it. The volume of petrol injected into a car is estimated in gallons, and the calories of assorted foods and drinks you drink are measured in calories. Since the body breaks down food in such a particular fashion, the amount of calories is a way to measure how much energy you'll receive from whatever you eat or drink. 'Calorie' is just another word for 'steam.'

Is It Real The Calories Are Harmful To You?

Calories aren't harmful to you, and they provide nutrients to the body. However, consuming a ton of calories and not losing enough of them by physical exercise will contribute to weight gain over time. Consuming minimal calories over time may prevent your body from functioning correctly, which can have a detrimental effect on your health. Foods such as lettuce contain relatively little calories (1 cup of shredded lettuce has fewer than ten calories), while peanuts have a ton of calories (1/2 cup of peanuts has 427 calories each day). Knowing how many calories your body needs per day will help you choose the best foods for you.

What Is Your Body's Calorie Utilization Process?

Simply to stay alive and work correctly, the body needs calories. This energy is used for essential tasks such as holding the heart pumping and breathing into your lungs. Calories are necessary for several primary and complex functions, including controlling body temperature and each cell's proper functioning in the human body. The more exercise you engage in, the more calories you can burn. Your body needs calories to expand and develop. You burn calories before you think about it, such as during food absorption, muscle regeneration during a workout, and sleeping.

How many calories are you looking for?

Since people are of various heights and have varying metabolisms, the number of calories they can ingest can vary depending on a range of reasons. These considerations include a person's size, age, weight, and amount of physical activity. The larger a person is, the more calories he or she will want, and vice versa. And if two people have the exact body dimensions, the number of calories they desire will vary due to how their bodies respond to what they consume. Calorie calculators are accessible on the internet and can determine the number of calories the body needs to be based on various factors. If you eat more calories than the body needs, the excess calories are stored as fat. If you eat fewer calories than you need, the body can switch to stored body fat for the energy it needs to survive. You can regulate your weight by understanding how many calories you like.

Basics in Macroeconomics

Carbohydrates, fats, and protein are known as macronutrients. These three nutrients, along with the term "macro," which means "big," are responsible for providing calories (the only other substance that provides calories is alcohol, which isn't a macronutrient, so we don't need it for survival). Those three macronutrients are broken down into all you consume. Your body doesn't recognize the food you eat as "poultry, sausage, potatoes, etc." Instead, anything you consume is categorized as starch, fat, or protein by the body. This is why these macronutrients are mentioned in large letters on every food or beverage product's nutrition mark.

What is a Carbohydrate?

Carbohydrates are the body's principal energy supply. Carbohydrates are divided into two types: complex and essential. A primary carbohydrate gives your body quick energy, but it doesn't last long. Since an elaborate carbohydrate takes longer to break down in your body, it provides a stable source of energy. Carbohydrates, both primary and complicated, are not detrimental to your body. Any of them may be beneficial to you during the day. When you wake up in the morning, it's possible that you haven't eaten anything in a previous couple of hours.

As a consequence, consuming easy carbs for quick energy is sometimes a brilliant idea. Complex carbohydrates are a perfect option for long-term stable life if you plan on staying away from home for a few hours. Consequently, incorporating both types of carbohydrates into your diet can help you better control your energy levels throughout the day.

Whole grains like whole wheat rye, oatmeal, and brown rice, and sweet potatoes and beans are examples of complex carbohydrates. Fruits, white bread, white rice, white potatoes, vegetables, juice, pop tarts, and other simple carbs are examples. Sugar is an essential carbohydrate and can be present in several different ways, including sugar, fructose, lactose, sucrose, etc. While all necessary and complex carbohydrates are broken down into glucose in the body, the main distinctions between the two are absorption and digestion.

What Is Protein?

When it comes to different cell roles in the body, protein helps develop and reconstruct tissue. It's an essential component for the growth of nails, hair, muscle, and other parts of the human body. Protein is made up of amino acids, which are the building blocks of the molecule. A whole protein comprises all 20 amino acids, while an imperfect protein lacks one or two amino acids. Complete proteins can be present in various foods, including pork, beef, seafood, legumes, milk, and whey protein. Incomplete proteins are found in foods such as rice, peas, nuts, and beans. For effective muscle growth, ingest at least 0.8 to 1.2 grams of protein per pound of body weight. Every specific protein is beneficial for developing and recovering tissue, regardless of the composition, absorption rate, or filtration process. There are variations between meat, fish, milk, legumes, soy, whey, and other protein sources, but any complex protein helps muscle repair and development. The most important thing is to get enough protein to meet your body's needs for optimal growth.

What Exactly Is Fat?

Fat regulates hormones, assists in cell transportation, and allows various nutrients to complete activities inside the body. Fat may also be a secondary source of nutrition for the body. If the body doesn't have enough carbohydrates readily accessible, it tends to fat as a nutrition source. Consequently, fat-burning aims to reduce the amount of primary energy (carbohydrates) consumed such that the body can use its secondary energy supply (body fat). Saturated fat, polyunsaturated fat, monounsaturated fat, and trans-fat are all forms of fat. Instead of the health benefits of trans-fat, it is advised that you stop it. Although each kind of fat has its own set of advantages and drawbacks, it's helpful to consider the total amount of fat in a particular product.

Peanut butter, oils, coconut, and almonds are examples of foods rich in fats. Low fat intake over time will trigger hormone levels to become unpredictable, so it's essential to consume enough fat even though you're trying to lose weight. Depending on the individual and health goal, the amount of fat needed daily could range from 15% to over 40% of total calories.

Weight-Loss or Weight-Gain Efficiency

You can lose weight while you are in a calorie deficiency, which means your body consumes more calories than you consume. This does not mean that you can lose any of your weight by burning fat. Lean mass, weight, and fat make up the body. This suggests that any weight lost or gained may originate from any of those three causes. You run the risk of losing weight if you lose fat, and you run the risk of adding fat if you add weight. Since you won't know how many calories you're consuming if you don't monitor your macros, you're more likely to lose muscle and add weight. Consuming the right amount of protein, fat, and carbohydrates will help you maintain power when losing weight and limit body fat gain while adding muscle.

Essential Nutrients

Food is a need of the human body. Your body will wither and decay if you don't feed. Not all food is deemed safe for the body, but certain foods are, and those are the foods you should eat. This collection of foods provides you with all of the health benefits that come from consuming food, as well as enough energy to help you live a productive life. So, here's a list of foods.

Fruits & Vegetables

The fruits are the first. Fruits are beneficial to the body and well-being. Fruit now has a wide variety of nutrients, from vitamins to fibers. Fibers aid in the digestive tract's proper functioning and support removing all anti-oxidants in the body. Bananas are a good source of potassium, fiber, and vitamins for the body. Avocados supply the body with both nutritious fats and non-harmful carbohydrates. Vitamin C and potassium are available in them. Berries, plums, peaches, pears, cherries, carrots, and watermelons are among the fruits you can consume. The fruit is abundant in vitamin C and assists in the elimination of contaminants from the body.

a dozen eggs

Eggs are the second item on the list, and they are a dietary powerhouse. They supply the body with a variety of nutrients that will aid in developing solid muscles and the vitamins and nutrients needed for better memory and the ability to carry out everyday tasks with ease. Eggs will also lower the risk of heart failure by supplying the body with the requisite cholesterol. They even help you shed weight and feel energized without reducing some vision loss.

Eggs are rich in vitamin B12, vitamin E, and selenium, improving the immune system. They ensure that you have a high immune system, which is helpful to your skin. Eggs may be consumed raw or cooked. Eggs unclog the clogs and reduce any infection that might be present in the body.

Meat, both red and white

Red and white meat are the following things to drink. Red meat is not advised, so if you do ingest it, do it in moderation so that the body receives the nutrients it needs. Since it contains much bioavailable iron, lean meat is the safest form of red meat to eat. Chicken breast is a good source of iron, and it's still a good source of white meat. Chicken breast is rich in nutrition and low in calories, which is good for the body. For a balanced body, lean meat is often advised.

Furthermore, grass-fed lamb meat is rich in omega-3 fatty acids, making it very safe for the body; nevertheless, unhealthy meat intake, particularly in large amounts, is not suitable for the body. As a consequence, you can eat meat in moderation.

Seeds and Nuts

Nuts and seeds are the following foods you can consume. Fiber, magnesium, and chia seed are also contained in almonds. They are rich in fiber, calcium, magnesium, and manganese, both essential nutrients for the body and good unsaturated fats. Nuts are abundant in fiber, which is helpful to the digestive tract. Peanuts are a non-nutrient snack that is high in antioxidants. Coconut oil supplies the body with essential fatty acids; however, nuts are high in calories and should be consumed cautiously. The majority of people love drinking them in abundance. It's not a brilliant idea to consume so much of them. Just enjoy them in moderation.

Fruits and vegetables

The crops are up next. There are several varieties of vegetables, but broccoli is the most common. Broccoli is a fiber-rich crop that lets the body absorb food properly. It also contains vitamin K and vitamin C, which the body needs. They're also high in protein. Carrots are rich in carotene and are an outstanding antioxidant that assists in eliminating toxins from the body. Cucumber is also an excellent crop to eat since it provides several vitamin K and nutrients and is low in carbohydrates and calories, and high in water. Cucumber has several nutrients that are beneficial for the body.

Tomatoes are high in vitamin C and potassium, and while they are classified as crops, they are technically fruits. You should eat several vegetables, including cabbage, tomatoes, broccoli, chili, and cauliflower. Many of these vegetables are highly useful to the human body.

garlic

Garlic is the next item on the list. Garlic includes the bioactive organic sulfur compound, which serves to strengthen the immune system. Garlic contains a variety of nutrients, including vitamin K and vitamin C. It also incorporates a lot of thread.

Veggies

The greens are up next. Greens are high in carbohydrates, but they are incredibly safe for the body, mainly if eaten as part of a high-carbohydrate diet. Brown rice is the perfect green to eat because it has a high amount of vitamin B1, magnesium, and fiber. The most common cereal is brown rice. Oats provide a lot of fiber called better hay, which has a lot of advantages. Quinoa supplies the body with nutrition and magnesium. It has a pleasant flavor and is prominent with health-conscious individuals.

a loaf of bread

The bread is the next thing on the list. The majority of white bread available in the area is heavily refined. It's challenging to find non-processed organic bread, but a healthy bread named Ezekiel bread is readily available. Several organically sprouted legumes and grains were used to produce Ezekiel bread. Low-carb bread made at home is another safe bread to eat. The most preferred kind of bread is bread cooked by average citizens and is likely to be better than factory-made bread.

Legume is a kind of legume.

Legumes are the next thing in the chart. Another food category that is highly recommended for its nutritious value is legumes. Kidney beans are legumes that provide adequate fiber, minerals, and vitamins to the body. It's best to prepare kidney beans thoroughly since they can be poisonous if eaten fresh. The unripe type of popular beans is green beans. Green beans are a common vegetable in Western countries. Lentils are a form of legume that is rich in fiber and the best plant-based protein source. However, it would help if you were mindful that legumes produce nutrients that impact digestive and nutrient absorption. As a consequence, you can soak legumes thoroughly before cooking and thoroughly cook them.

Milk and Dairy Products

Dairy items are the next item on the list. Dairy goods are well-known for their vital calcium and magnesium content, all of which are beneficial to the bones and teeth. Obesity and type 2 diabetes have been linked to full-fat dairy. Grass-fed dairy products are more healthy than factory-made dairy products, and they produce a lot of vitamin K2 and by-active acid. Cheese is rich in nutrition, has the same number of nutrients as a whole cup of milk, and is tasty.

Whole milk provides a variety of vitamins and nutrients and a lot of protein from animals. Yogurt includes live colonies that are good for the body and a lot of healthy bacteria. They, like milk, offer a range of health benefits to the body. Skim milk is rich in calcium, which is essential for healthy bones, protein, and vitamin D. Since skim milk has no saturated fat, it is advised that you consume it three times a day.

Oil and Fats

The following subject is fat and gasoline. A ton of fats and oils are deemed safe for you. Vitamin K2 is available in fat butter made from grass-fed cows. Coconut oil is beneficial to the body, especially when attempting to lose belly fat. Extra virgin olive oil is one of the healthiest vegetable oils available. It produces a high number of antioxidants, rendering it heart-friendly, as well as mono-saturated fats. It is beneficial to eat fat and oil, so you should be careful how much you consume because consuming so much puts the body at risk for high blood pressure, heart disease, and diabetes.

Apple Cider Vinegar is a vinegar made from apples.

Apple cider vinegar is the next thing in the chart. Apple cider vinegar has a wide range of health benefits. It assists weight control by lowering blood sugar levels in the body. One of the healthiest weight-loss guidelines is apple cider vinegar. It helps in the rejuvenation of lubrication. It will assist in processing synovial fluid, which is used to lubricate the joints if you have joint complications. You may use vinegar to produce meals and salad dressings.

Foods from the Shore

Seafood is the next thing in the chart. Seafood contains all seafood and non-fishy family members. The bulk of edible seafood falls from the fish and non-fish families. Omega-3 fatty acids are found in most diets, but having them will help you live longer. They also lower the chances of developing illnesses like schizophrenia and depression. They also aid in the improvement of brain performance and cognitive performance. Any fish has a standard nutritional profile; tuna shrimp, sardines, and salmon are excellent examples of seafood to consume.

Beans are a legume.

Beans are the next item on the menu. Beans are strong in fiber and plant-based nutrition. Vitamins, minerals, copper, iron, and vitamin B are also abundant in them. Beans are available in several types, including spaghetti, salad broth, and curry, as well as baked goods. Beans include disease-fighting phytochemicals that shield cells from the destruction associated with colon cancer.

Chocolate (dark)

Dark chocolate is the next item on the list. Dark chocolate is renowned not only for its delicious flavor but also for its health benefits. Cocoa is used to produce dark chocolate, and cocoa is abundant in antioxidants. Four servings of dark chocolate, eaten at least four days a week, will tend to strengthen your blood vessels and increase your blood pressure. Dark chocolate helps to keep the body's processes in check.

Benefits of a Healthy Body

It is essential to sustain a balanced body to live a long and healthy existence. A healthier body allows you to live a more active and prosperous existence, which leads to more extraordinary accomplishments and the ability to mature gracefully. To sustain a healthy body, one must eat healthy food, indulge in daily exercise, keep a stress-free mind, get adequate sleep, and enjoy a healthy lifestyle. Below are ten influential factors to hold your body in decent condition.

Immune System Booster

A safe body ensures that all of the body's functions are running well and that all of the necessary antibodies for battling disease are formed in sufficient quantities. The body would be able to combat infections and prevent itself from being ill in this manner. Even if the body is incapable of battling all conditions, a safe body is more prone to fend off most seasonal diseases than a sick body. However, once the body's immune system deteriorates, it is essential to stop eating alcohol and sugary foods and beverages, as microbes have a strong preference for sugar.

Reduces the likelihood of developing some cancer

According to a biological description, cancer is described as unregulated cell division caused by a mutation in cells' DNA. DNA is in charge of instructing cells about where to split, how many cells to divide, and how to fix compromised cells; as the cells' DNA mutates, the cells fragment uncontrollably and fail to execute cancer's required functions. DNA mutations may be transmitted naturally, biologically predisposed by chemicals that induce illness or induced by harmful habits such as inadequate nutrition, smoking, heavy alcohol intake, and obesity. The leading cause of the disease is an unsafe lifestyle. Standard DNA is present in a healthy body, ensuring that cell division and repair are also regulated. As a result, maintaining a balanced body is essential.

Increases the sum of energy in the body

A balanced body has a lot of potentials, and it has worked hard to get there. A balanced diet is essential for good health. A balanced diet provides the body with the minerals, sugars, and proteins it needs. Exercising allows the body to respond to rough care, and as a result, each workout session renders the organization more efficient than ever. A decent night's sleep clears the subconscious and relieves exhaustion. As a consequence of this collection, the authority has a higher degree of energy and is more efficient.

Reduces the likelihood of infertility

Being overweight or underweight will make things more challenging to conceive. Infertility may also be exacerbated by the usage of recreational medications and smoke. Men that are overweight, smoke, or drink a lot of alcohol have lower sperm counts, which leads to infertility. Infertility may be caused by both being underweight and being overweight in women. All of the above conditions are the product of a sick body. Consequently, eating better to stop becoming underweight, walking to reduce obesity and overweight situations, living a balanced lifestyle, and preserving a healthy body will assist with infertility therapy.

Stroke and heart-related problems are avoided.

A stroke happens when the brain is deprived of oxygen for a prolonged time, culminating in cell death. Oxygen deprivation can be induced by a blockage or rupture of an artery, resulting in the leakage of oxygenated blood that keeps cells alive and well. Fat accumulation, which prevents the proper distribution of blood to the brain, is one of the blocked arteries' triggers. Unhealthy diets and depression can also be factors. Heart attacks and coronary artery disease are two severe heart conditions. Coronary artery disorder is triggered by so much cholesterol obstructing the body's blood flow. The coronary artery's rapture causes a heart attack, which occurs as the heart pumps blood at a more significant rhythmic pressure than average. Increases the strain on the highway, allowing it to tear.

According to experts, exercising, living a balanced lifestyle, getting adequate rest, avoiding fatigue, and eating a healthy diet are the safest treatments for both illnesses. Doctors emphasize the importance of maintaining our bodies well to combat diseases such as cardiac disease and stroke.

Enhances a few career options

Athletes in sports must uphold a high quality of life as well as an outstanding physical appearance. Athletes must observe a strict diet, workout daily, get adequate sleep, and, most notably, abstain from using illegal substances and drinking excessive alcohol quantities. Models and dancers in the film sector are now expected to stick to certain living conditions. These safe expectations mean that their bodies are in decent shape and will continue to succeed in their professions.

Enhances Longevity

A long-term study has demonstrated that maintaining a balanced body guarantees a long existence. Exercising for as little as twenty minutes a day decreased the likelihood of dying prematurely. Suitable lifestyle modifications, such as proper eating, are often crucial for maintaining a long life. Particularly at an early age, a stable body helps one conduct activities that would be impossible if they were ill or deceased. It also ensures that more time will be spent with families. Grandparents are eager to see and bond with their grandchildren because they have their bodies in decent condition.

Assists in weight management

A balanced body has been accomplished by good body care and exercise. And if you don't want to lose weight, having a good quality of life can eventually contribute to healthier body weight. Maintaining a balanced bodyweight needs a routine regimen of a few hours of exercise and proper nutrition. As a flat body product, the body can have an excellent immune system, reduce heart failure, and raise body energy levels.

Enhances Moods and Emotions

According to a report, exercising our bodies helps us feel comfortable and content. It is triggered by the release of endorphins, which are chemicals released by brain cells. Exercising guarantees that one maintains an athletic physique, which implies that one's image can strengthen, resulting in greater self-confidence. We exist in a society where disappointments and disasters are commonplace. It's essential to hold our bodies in top shape for better mental control and cognitive performance.

Aids in the Management of Diabetes

Type one diabetes happens when the body attacks the body's insulin-producing cells. Type two diabetes occurs when the body destroys its insulin-producing cells. Then he or she would have to rely on insulin shots for the rest of his or her life. When the body cannot consume sugar from the blood and turn it into energy for the cells, it is known as type two diabetes. Tier 1 diabetes is caused by unhealthy working environments, a lack of exercise, and a poor diet. Early signs of diabetes, such as pre-diabetes and gestational diabetes, can be controlled through a balanced diet and exercise. Maintaining a balanced body involves regulating body insulin balance and reducing diabetes-related deaths such as elevated blood pressure, heart disease, renal failure, and blood vessel hardening.

Improves the memory of the brain

A balanced body necessitates a healthy diet, which includes all of the dietary nutrients. Vitamins are among these nutrients. Vitamins, especially vitamins C, E, and D, and Omega 3 fatty acids and flavonoids, are essential for developing a brain with a strong memory. A nutritious diet can also aid in the prevention of dementia and cognitive loss. Dementia is defined by a lack of awareness and impairments of one's capacity to communicate, remember, or even solve problems. Dementia that is not induced by severe damage to the brain will be minimized by consuming a regular diet.

Both the bones and the teeth are strengthened.

Teeth and bone structure may be improved by maintaining a balanced body. Three servings of dairy products a day are indicated for calcium. The body must therefore be subjected to physical workouts, the most common of which is lifting weights. A balanced diet is also essential. For stronger teeth and muscles, calcium and magnesium-rich foods must be eaten. Calcium is abundant in particular cereals, while magnesium is abundant in legumes, berries, whole grains, and beans.

Boosts Self-Confidence

Getting a sound body is one of the causes of poor self-esteem. We exist in a culture that is complex and full of varying fashion tastes. Everyone wishes to look healthy, but our bodies will let us down at times, which can be harmful to our self-esteem. This, though, can be improved, and our self-esteem can be enhanced in no time. A proper diet and daily body workouts, and keeping a stable mind by rest and thought management would be a good start. It takes time to see results, so if you do, you'll have a good body. This is equivalent to destroying two birds with one stone in that one will improve their self-confidence by enhancing their looks and still gain a state of wellbeing by maintaining a healthier body.

A Balanced Body improves better Sleep

People who have dysfunctional bodies also have a tough time sleeping. Obese people appear to sweat a lot and have difficulty breathing when sleeping. Healthy people sleep well and have no respiratory issues when asleep. Exercising the body means that the body's systems operate efficiently and that extra fats are burned out, resulting in overnight sweating. A balanced body may also be accomplished by eating correctly and preventing drug and alcohol misuse. A safe body contributes to a decent night's sleep.

Chapter 10; keto diet and weight loss

A "typical" ketogenic diet includes at least 70% of calories from fat, less than 10% from carbohydrates, and less than 20% from protein. According to the American Epilepsy Society, the ketogenic diet needs 90 percent of daily calories to come from fat. The sum of carbohydrates or carbohydrates differs as much as there are 4 grams of fat for any combined 1 gram of carb and protein. Cheese, butter, cheese, almonds, fish, pork, olive oil, and non-starchy vegetables such as broccoli, cauliflower, greens, and spinach will aid. Apps and online programs will do the algebra for you if you're arithmetic impaired. (Regardless, the keto diet varies significantly from the USDA's dietary guidelines, which allow for carbohydrates to account for 45 to 65 percent of total calories, fat to account for 20 to 35 percent, and protein to account for 10 to 35 percent.)

The ketogenic diet helps to place you in a state of ketosis by boosting your fat metabolism. In a ketogenic condition, the body burns fat for energy rather than carbs, and fats may be transformed to ketones to power the body while glucose levels are inadequate.

Per day, an average adult must consume less than 20 to 50 grams of net carbohydrates (total carbs minus fiber) to maintain ketosis. It's easy to get across the line: a thick slice of bread contains 21 carbohydrates, a medium apple contains 25, and a cup of milk contains 12. Carla Prado, an assistant professor and head of the University of Alberta's Human Nutrition Research Unit, said, "It's very limiting." Bread and drink are off-limits, but so are high-sugar fruits and starchy vegetables like potatoes, as well as excessive protein. Dieters must still be on the lookout for secret carbohydrates, which are frequently undetectable to the naked eye but coat the seemingly keto-friendly fried cheese.

Is it possible to lose weight on the keto diet?

Yeah, indeed. That tends to be the case in the short term. According to a recent literature analysis of low-carb diets published by the National Lipid Association, a low-carbohydrate diet will help you lose more weight over the first two to six months than a regular high-carbohydrate, low-fat diet.

Carol F. Kirkpatrick, director of Idaho State University's Wellness Center and lead author of the latest literature review, said, "By 12 months, the benefit is effectively gone."

Following that, weight reduction tends to be similar between the two standard diet programs. She claims that keto is better used to kick-start a diet while switching to a carb level that can be sustained over time.

When it comes to the keto diet, how long would it take to achieve results?

It's the promised land in diets for others. Instead of dreading carrot sticks, they should eat chorizo and scrambled eggs guilt-free. Some research shows that while people are in ketosis, they are less hungry and have fewer cravings.

Dr. Mackenzie C. Cervenka, medical director of Johns Hopkins Hospital's Adult Epilepsy Diet Center, said, "That's why it's been so common with the general public." "Because it's easy to adhere to until you're in ketosis." According to physicians, it typically takes one to four days to reach the state. However, this depends on several variables, including activity level: a runner, for example, can sprint there quicker than a couch potato.

The ketogenic diet tends to show fast results: The first few pounds might seem to be falling away. That may be alluring, but it's most definitely just water weight. So it's down to energy in minus energy out, according to dietitians. According to Dr. Linsenmeyer, who is also the head of Saint Louis University's

Didactic Curriculum in Dietetics, you can gain weight on any diet if you eat 5,000 calories a day.

She explained, "It's not because it'll magically shift your metabolism, so the calories don't count anymore." When the carbohydrates are resumed, the water weight recovers.

Will the ketogenic diet, on the other hand, help you consume more calories?

There is some proof to confirm this. Here, too, the analysis is minimal and contradictory. It may be a minor impact that has little bearing on weight loss. According to one report, this is the case. For two months, 17 obese or overweight volunteers were placed in metabolic wards and had every spoonful food tracking. (To be explicit regarding the topics of scientific experiments, this recounting of the science utilizes definitional words like "obese.") They ate a high-carb diet for the first month and a ketogenic diet for the second, with all programs containing the same amount of calories.

Kevin Hall, integrative physiology section head for the National Institute of Diabetes and Digestive and Kidney Diseases' Laboratory of Biological Modeling, said, "We feed them every morsel of food that they ate." "There were no days off." In the end, while the participants' insulin levels dropped as they ate the bunless burger, they didn't lose much more weight than when they ate the breaded burger. However, the analysis was constrained by restricted sample size and the absence of a placebo group on the back-to-back regimens.

A low-carb diet can cater to some people. According to a survey that tracked 609 overweight people for a year on either a low-carb or low-fat diet, diet isn't superior. According to a randomized controlled study that looked at a low-carb diet that was less stringent than the keto diet, all participants dropped about the same amount of weight — between 12 to 13 pounds on average. What is the takeaway message? "You should excel on both," said Christopher Gardner, the study's lead author and a Stanford Prevention Science Center professor of medicine and diet scientist.

Is there any long-term advantage of the ketogenic diet?

It is also unknown. Dr. Prado of the University of Alberta, who co-authored a narrative study on the ketogenic diet as a potential cancer treatment, said, "If you advise people to go on this diet indefinitely and over a prolonged period, there is little evidence."

Children with epilepsy benefit from the diet: Within six months on the regimen, about a third or two-thirds of patients had 50% fewer seizures. (Epilepsy was treated by eating as early as 400 B.C.) The ketogenic diet is nearly a century old, having first achieved traction as a cure for epilepsy before developing an anticonvulsant drug.) While there are case reports about how ten patients with an uncommon disorder did on a diet over a decade, several well-designed studies in this area have only lasted two years.

Is a low-carb diet beneficial to people with diabetes?

Yeah, indeed. "Carbohydrate is the most important driver of blood sugar," said Duke's Dr. Yancy, who believes the food will benefit those with diabetes.

A recent randomized research study involved 263 people with Type 2 diabetes in community care appointments, half receiving drug adjustments for improved blood sugar regulation and the other half getting low-carb diet weight loss therapy. (All of the study's subjects have a BMI that was either overweight or obese.) According to results reported in the Journal of the American Medical Association Internal Medicine, all groups had lower overall blood sugar levels after 48 weeks. The weight loss party on the low-carb diet, on the other hand, lost more weight, used less insulin, and reported less dangerous low blood sugar events.

A low-carbohydrate diet seems to raise normal blood sugar levels of Type 2 diabetes patients faster than a high-carbohydrate, low-fat diet in the first year. The National Lipid Association finds that during that time frame, the disparity nearly vanishes — but for one significant benefit: the low-carb participants were willing to use fewer drugs. Dr. Yancy explained, "People like it, and they don't like being on diabetes medications."

Is there a way to consume more fat in a safe way?

Dr. Cervenka of Johns Hopkins Hospital doesn't rule out saturated fats from animal products as she begins her epilepsy patients with a low-carbohydrate diet. She needs them to get used to the latest food habits. However, if their cholesterol levels start to increase, she suggests transitioning to foods and oils high in mono- and polyunsaturated fats, such as avocados or olive oil.

Although the impact of the diet on LDL ("bad") cholesterol seems to be mixed, a study by the National Lipid Association showed that a relatively low-carbohydrate diet appears to boost HDL cholesterol (commonly known as the good cholesterol). Similar to weight reduction, it seems that these effects do not extend for a year. Only lower triglyceride amounts tend to be long-lasting. Other findings: The data on blood pressure is mixed, and increased mental clarity claims aren't backed up by research.

What effect does all that fatty meat have on your health?

What happens, for example, if you remove bananas, legumes, and whole grains from your diet, both of which have been related to lower cardiometabolic risk in studies?

Dr. Neil J. Stone, a preventive cardiologist at Northwestern University's Feinberg School of Medicine, is concerned about this since several of his keto diet patients' insufficient cholesterol levels have skyrocketed. (It doesn't happen to everybody. However, it does to some.) "Any diet that increases significant coronary heart disease risk factors puts patients at risk in the long run," he added.

(There's still a lot of discussion around LDL particles and whether the firm that's growing with the keto diet, bigger LDL particles, increases the risk of heart disease.)

According to an American Heart Association guideline co-authored by Dr. Stone, reducing dietary saturated fat, such as fatty meats and high-fat dairy, may help. Swapping it out for unsaturated fats like safflower or olive oil can lower your risk of heart disease. Still, before embarking on some diet, he suggests that you remember the following: What are your objectives? Are they temporary or permanent? Is it feasible to get there without taking as many chances?

EASY KETO BREAKFAST RECIPES

Sheet Pan Pancakes (15 servings)

- The perfect make-ahead keto pancake recipe. It's so much easier than flipping pancakes in a skillet, and it makes 15 servings. It freezes well, too, so you can stretch them out to last for several weeks!
- 221 calories, 18.7g fat, 7.5g carbs, 4.2g fiber, 7.5g protein
- Add 1 tbsp butter to round out the meal: Adds 102 calories, 7g fat, 0g carbs, 0g fiber, 0g protein

Sheet Pan Frittata (8 servings)

- Another leisurely sheet pan breakfast that helps you prep for the week ahead. Cut it into servings and store it in a covered container in the fridge.
- 284 calories, 20.6g fat, 3.7g carbs, 0.7g fiber, 16.5g protein
- Add 1/4 avocado to round out the meal: Adds 81 calories, 7.3g fat, 4.2g carbs, 1.3g fiber, 1g protein

Cinnamon Crunch Cereal (6 servings)

- Easy to make and egg-free, this tasty keto cereal recipe makes a beautiful breakfast, but it's also great for snacking. Make ahead and store in an airtight container on the counter for up to a week.
- 257 calories, 24.5g fat, 6.5g carbs, 3.4g fiber, 4.6g protein
- Add 2 tbsp heavy whipping cream to round out the meal: Adds 58 calories, 6g of fat, 1g carbs, 0g fiber, 0.8g protein

Avocado Green Tea Smoothie (2 servings)

- This unusual flavor combination works and is packed with antioxidants. Best of all, it's the kind of breakfast you can whip up in a matter of minutes.
- 229 calories, 16.7g fat, 4.4g carbs, 2.9g fiber, 14.1g protein
- Add two slices of bacon to round out the meal: Adds 86 calories, 6.7g fat, 0g carbs, 0g fiber, 6g protein

EASY KETO DINNER RECIPES

Chicken and Broccoli Casserole (6 servings)

- Creamy one-pan deliciousness! If you grab a rotisserie chicken, this delicious keto casserole is so easy to make and comes together in 25 minutes. And the leftovers reheat well.
- 493 calories, 34.7g fat, 6.1g carbs, 1.5g fiber, 27g protein

Asian Steak Bites (6 servings)

- Quick-cooking steak bites are a great way to divvy up a nice sirloin for several servings. Marinate the steak bites before you head to work, and it will take you only about 10 minutes to make this easy meal.
- 280 calories, 16.9g fat, 2.5g carbs, 0g fiber, 23.1g protein
- Add some cauliflower rice to round out the meal. If it's sautéed in a few tbsp of butter, it will add about 80 calories, 5.6g fat, 4g carbs, 2g fiber, and 2g protein.
- Other sides to consider roasted broccoli, small green salad, sautéed zucchini noodles.

Mexican Cauliflower Rice (6 servings)

- One of my most popular keto dinner recipes, and it's your whole meal in one pan. It takes 25 minutes, start to finish, and kids love it too.
- 352 calories, 21.7g fat, 7g carbs, 2g fiber, 29.1g protein
- Top with 1 tbsp sour cream and about 1/8 of avocado: Adds 64 calories, 6.1g fat, 2.4g carbs, 0.6g fiber, 0.7g protein

Sheet Pan Chicken and Veggies (6 servings)

- Notice a trend here? Sheet pans are great for easy cooking and meal prep, and this delicious one-pan dinner is proof!
- 437 calories, 29.4g fat, 8.8g carbs, 3.5g fiber, 29.4g protein

Garlic Butter Salmon (4 servings)

- Yup, you guessed it, another easy sheet pan meal! Feel accessible to sub broccoli or green beans in for the cauliflower to shake things up a bit.
- 450 calories, 23.8g fat, 6.3g carbs, 2.4g fiber, 36.9g protein

Air Fryer Pork Chops (4 servings)

- Tender and juicy, with a delectable browned butter sage sauce. Don't worry if you don't have an air fryer, as I have also included stovetop instructions.
- 485 calories, 30.5g fat, 0.7g carbs, 0g fiber, 46.7g protein
- Add a small green salad and 2 tbsp of your choice of keto salad dressing to round out the meal: Adds about 115 calories, 8g fat, 5g carbs, 1.5g fiber, 2g protein (depending on the dressing).

SNACKS AND DESSERTS

Cream of Mushroom Soup with Brown Butter (4 servings)

- Super creamy and with only five ingredients, it's a keto newbie's dream recipe. So simple to make and so much flavor, it's a great snack or light lunch.
- 198 calories, 17.7g fat, 4.6g carbs, 0.6g fiber, 4.6g protein

Keto Peppermint Patties (12 servings)

- Simple dairy-free treats can help conquer craving for something sweet and keep you from giving in to the high carb junk.
- 126 calories, 13.6g fat, 2.9g carbs, 1.4g fiber, 0.4g protein

Keto Butter Pecan Cookies (10 servings)

- These viral cookies are so easy to make and are a delightful keto snack. No one can ever believe that they are low carb and sugar-free.
- 240 calories, 22.3g fat, 5.3g carbs, 3.1g fiber, 5g protein

www.ingramcontent.com/pod-product-compliance
Lightning Source LLC
Chambersburg PA
CBHW031347060726

47590CB00007B/2659